An Introduction to Medical
Dance/Movement Therapy

of related interest

Music Therapy and Neurological Rehabilitation
Performing Health
Edited by David Aldridge
ISBN 1 84310 302 8

The Healing Flow: Artistic Expression in Therapy
Creative Arts and the Process of Healing: An Image/Word
Approach Inquiry
Martina Schnetz
ISBN 1 84310 205 6

Medical Art Therapy with Adults
Edited by Cathy Malchiodi
ISBN 1 85302 679 4

Medical Art Therapy with Children
Edited by Cathy Malchiodi
ISBN 1 85302 677 8

Using Voice and Movement in Therapy
The Practical Application of Voice Movement Therapy
Paul Newham
ISBN 1 85302 592 5

Authentic Movement
Essays by Mary Starks Whitehouse, Janet Adler and
Joan Chodorow
Edited by Patrizia Pallaro
ISBN 1 85302 653 0

An Introduction to Medical Dance/Movement Therapy
Health Care in Motion

Sharon W. Goodill

Foreword by John Graham-Pole

Jessica Kingsley Publishers
London and Philadelphia

First published in 2005
by Jessica Kingsley Publishers
116 Pentonville Road
London N1 9JB, UK
and
400 Market Street, Suite 400
Philadelphia, PA 19106, USA

www.jkp.com

Copyright © Sharon W. Goodill 2005
Foreword copyright © John Graham-Pole 2005
Front cover image © Cheryl Mitchell Downer

Library of Congress Cataloging in Publication Data

Goodill, S. (Sherry)
    An introduction to medical dance/movement therapy : health care in motion / Sharon W. Goodill ; foreword by John Graham-Pole.-- 1st American pbk. ed.
        p. cm.
    Includes bibliographical references and index.
    ISBN 1-84310-785-6 (pbk.)
    1. Dance therapy. I. Title.
    RM931.D35G66 2005
    615.8'5155--dc22

                                                                    2004017937

British Library Cataloguing in Publication Data
A CIP catalogue record for this book is available from the British Library

ISBN-13: 978 1 84310 785 9
ISBN-10: 1 84310 785 6

Printed and Bound in Great Britain by
Athenaeum Press, Gateshead, Tyne and Wear

Contents

List of figures

Foreword

This millennium has laid down the gauntlet of choice for all who serve others, as mothers and fathers, grandparents and grandchildren, as teachers and politicians, healers and pastoral carers, as social and psychological therapists. We can hold back our judgments, can listen, watch, hone our senses, link our genius with humanity's original genius, and dance together. Or we can strut our stuff briefly on life's stage, satiate our egos as performers, then, seeing nothing much changed, give in to cynicism and despair at our collective human plight, our helplessness to reverse the tide.

The choice is simple, but far from easy. Art as psychotherapy, art as medicine, shows us a way, arguably *the* way.

I confess to being less than objective on the subject of dance. If your body moves, if it vibrates, it dances. When this is the subject, there can be no object: life, everyone's life is dance. The problem is, most of us have forgotten this; forgotten consciously how to dance. Granted, we cannot stop oscillating at a cellular level; but it has become indecent to show our cellular selves. Some say, perhaps, decency at all costs, however high those costs become.

For they are surely high enough; at risk is the sacrifice of our human authenticity and grace. It takes an utterly conscious effort to reclaim it; but reclaim it we must to live our divine truths. What can I say to you, Sharon Goodill, but thank you for your graceful and authentic efforts?

You are deeply compassionate in acknowledging how understandable such helplessness is; understandable but of no use to our survival. To this challenge you offer the antidote of the dance. Let the dance lead us, in faith that our innate skills remain untarnished, stand at attention ready to move, to meet and fulfill every requisite of our work of service.

So you extend your hands to us, offer to lead us back onto the universal dance floor. If we would rather die than expose ourselves to public gaze, nevertheless you remain inspired and undiscouraged. You have sought to teach us, every two-left-footed one among us, step by step, cadence by cadence, measure by measure, to "trip it as we go," to slow the tempo and attend, to feel, hear, and see, the full diversity of human oscillation. You delicately require of us that we tap into our cellular memories and uncover the shy place of unity that promises to bring forth human harmony in its wake.

Your scholarship is rigorous, runs wide and deep. You claim it is not exhaustive, yet your comprehensive synthesis of dance/movement therapy (DMT) has located and sourced 100 journals, 200 books and 150 websites, theses and dissertations, at least. You range from an explication of the theoretical base of DMT, through its successes in America and beyond, to your future vision of its evolution in education and research. How exciting to see its emergence from the strictly mental health field to its application to primarily physical ailments, in morphic resonance with the evolution of the more established language, musical, visual and dramatic arts therapies over the past twenty years. Your body of work emerges from the heart of health psychology; and the world is hungry for it.

You take a practical bent, as any dynamic work must, with vignettes, exercises and interviews from your own and others' experience in this field as well as the much larger ones of medicine, neuroscience, nursing and psychology. Your writing is elegant, assured and provocative. And what a wise choice to make your home base for this adventure Jessica Kingsley Publishers, a house of the highest repute for bringing us the spectrum of humanities wedded to humanity, of art in the service of human reemergence.

I am happy to know you; am moved by the deepest gratitude for the gift of your book, this "Project Demonstrating Excellence," and for the emergence of your intellectual studies, and you yourself, into a larger world. Thank God for it.

John Graham-Pole MBBS MRCP MD
October 2004

Preface

It was just over a decade ago when David Eisenberg's acclaimed study out of Harvard unearthed the fact that millions of Americans spend billions of unreimbursed health care dollars yearly on complementary and alternative therapies (Eisenberg *et al.* 1993). This news, and the society's renewed interest in the mind/body connection and body oriented therapies, created opportunities for dance/movement therapy (DMT) in the modern arenas of wellness and in medical settings. I was drawn into this in 1993, with the fortunate awarding of a research grant from the newly formed Office of Alternative Medicine at the National Institute of Health (NIH). I learned that there was a legacy of DMT work with medical patients, and a strong interest among dance/movement therapists in this application.

It seems timely to gather together in one place the creative and interesting work with medical patients in our field, and this book is the first known publication with that specific purpose. The many examples, projects, studies, written and presented works, when amassed, suggest that there is indeed a discernible specialty of the profession, which I presume to call "medical dance/movement therapy." In using this descriptor, I am simply following two of our sister specialties in the creative arts therapies: art and music therapy, where several volumes on their medical specializations have been published.

My method for researching the book could best be described as systematic literature review. This involves locating, surveying, organizing and synthesizing the known and available studies in a discipline or topic area. The primary domain includes clinical work, research and thinking within the field of DMT. For this, the literature was supplemented by a series of interviews with dance/movement therapists who have focused their work on medical populations. For coverage of the relevant domains outside the DMT literature, I made several choices about scope and topic, based mostly on my own experiences working in an academic health care system for several years. Having observed the success of health psychology in general health care, I turned to theory and research in that discipline for several constructs and approaches that might be useful in our thinking. Then, because of the primacy of the mind/body connection in DMT, I brought in scientific information that links physiology with behavior and with internal, subjective states. In all areas, I sought to bring into the light useful and interesting work that may not yet be well known to most dance/movement therapists.

This text represents a first attempt at describing this specialized work and giving it a theoretical context. In addition to telling the stories of medical DMT, I have included a number of richly applicable concepts from related fields, and indicated some potent future directions for the development of medical DMT. I have not attempted to weave all these components together to construct a distinct and cohesive theory of medical DMT. It would be premature, and possibly inappropriate, to propose a new model or framework at this time. This work is still emerging. Thus, this volume can be considered descriptive and pre-theoretical. It lays out some building blocks, articulates some hypotheses, and leaves the dialogue open for theory development in the future.

Acknowledgments

This textbook represents the culmination of study for a Ph.D. in medical psychology with a concentration in mind/body studies. I have come to this point only with the help and support of many people in my personal and professional life. My gratitude goes first to my remarkable "team" of doctoral committee advisors: Bill McKelvie EdD, and Ira Fritz PhD, of The Union Institute and University, Mario Rodriguez PhD, Robyn Flaum Cruz PhD, Winnie Hohlt PhD, and Carolyn Gordon PhD. They all found the perfect balance of challenge and encouragement – my accomplishment here is testimony to their gifts as teachers and guides.

The inspiration of my colleagues and friends in dance/movement therapy (DMT) brought me to this project. I am deeply and forever grateful to my mentor, Dianne Dulicai, for her belief in me and her exemplary living. The five therapists interviewed for this book entrusted me with the telling of their superb clinical work, and for their time and confidence I am most grateful. Susan Kierr also generously provided excerpts from her unpublished manuscripts on medical DMT work. Two leaders in medical DMT stand out: Susan Cohen and Ilene Serlin. Their clinical work, teachings and writings have provided a model on which I have based my own. I truly believe that without them, we would not be able to claim or define medical DMT as a specialty in the field.

Thanks are due to several others who enriched and supported my doctoral work in meaningful ways. To the courageous and visionary people of the Wellness Community Delaware I am indebted, especially to Program Director Sean Hebbel. My amazing co-workers at Drexel University listened, advised, questioned, and picked up a good deal of work I've left undone: Gayle Gates, Ellen Schelly Hill, Paul Nolan, Gail Wells, Nancy Gerber (my learning partner at The Union Institute and University) and especially Ron Hays, who provided the space and time for this work to be completed. The participants in two pilots of a medical DMT course, in Tel Aviv and in Philadelphia, gave me a chance to try out much of what is in this volume and brought their own fruitful thoughts to the process.

Personal support from a host of loving friends and family members formed the bedrock from which I've worked. The friendship of Mary and Mandell Much, Julie Ritter, Nancy Contel, Cheryl Downer and my sister Virginia Barnhart have sustained me throughout—to say nothing of the help with childrearing and transportation. In every way imaginable my loving husband John Goodill, who is my wind and my anchor, inspired and enabled this pursuit. Our very beautiful daughters, Libbie and Claire, have waited a long time for the completion of this project, and I am humbly grateful for their patience and their pride.

Part I

Overview

CHAPTER 1

Introduction

So embrace your chance
And join our Dance
Our dance of alchemy
Where dreams and fears
And pain and years
Dissolve in synergy

From "Dance of Alchemy" by R.A. Lippin[1]

Purpose and scope of the book

The aim of this volume is to describe the emerging application of dance/ movement therapy, a creative arts therapy, to the needs of those with a primary medical illness. There are three main objectives for this text:

1. to define the subspecialty of medical dance/movement therapy

2. to ground the clinical application in theoretical and scientific discoveries from related fields of health psychology and the medical sciences, and

3. to encourage research on and increased utilization of medical dance/movement therapy in general health care systems.

---

[1] Reproduced from *The Arts in Psychotherapy,* 7, R. A. Lippin, "Dance of Alchemy" pp.273–4, 1980, with permission from Elsevier.

To date, this book represents the first known attempt to compile, synthesize and publish the work that has been done with medical populations by dance/movement therapists.

I hope that this book will interest dance/movement therapy professionals and students as well as health care professionals who collaborate with, supervise, or initiate dance/movement therapy programming. Others who are interested in mind/body approaches to health and healing will also find the book of interest.

Dance/movement therapy (DMT) is formally defined as "the psychotherapeutic use of movement as a process which furthers the emotional, cognitive, social and physical integration of the individual" (American Dance Therapy Association n.d.). DMT is a specialty discipline in the mental health field, along with the other creative arts therapies (art, music, drama, poetry and psychodrama therapies). Academically, the field combines and synthesizes the study of psychological and social processes with other theoretical constructs from both the art of movement and kinesiological/biological principles of movement. Clinically, the work comprises a mind/body integrated approach to psychotherapy. Both the client(s) and the therapist attend to and address the sensed, kinesthetic and motoric connections between cognitive processes (including the creative process), emotional responses, interactional patterns and the issues relevant to the therapy. Common objectives of this therapy are, in part:

- increased integration of cognitive, affective and physical experience

- expressive competence

- increased self-awareness.

Assessment and clinical techniques are both sophisticated and flexible, so the therapy is adapted to the needs of a broad range of populations. Dance/movement therapists emphasize the congruence and connections between the verbal and nonverbal modes of expression. However, assessment and therapy can proceed entirely in the nonverbal realm of movement, touch, rhythm and spatial interactions, and so the approach is well suited to the needs of people who cannot participate in verbally oriented forms of psychotherapy. In addition, principles and techniques borrowed from this form of clinical interaction can also inform and enhance the work of other health care professionals by increasing sensitivity to these subjective, sensed components of the patient's condition, and by improving the patient–caregiver relationship through better communication skills in the nonverbal dimension.

Since the establishment of DMT as a professional discipline in the United States in 1966, most of the work of dance/movement therapists has taken place in mental health and special education settings. Nonetheless, there is a longstanding interest among dance/movement therapists in working with those who are primarily medically ill, with theoretical and clinical explorations dating back to the 1970s. Evidence of this interest and emerging expertise is abundant. For example, several articles have been written in peer-reviewed academic journals over the last decade, and a handful of funded research projects on medical applications of DMT have been conducted (including one by this author). Dozens of Master's theses have explored concepts and applications of DMT with medical populations and numerous professional conference presentations have been given on these topics (Ascheim *et al.* 1992; Cannon *et al.* 1997). Recent scientific advances from various branches of basic and clinical medical science provide explanatory models for the processes underlying DMT, and the DMT community has been increasingly engaged in discussion and collaborations with this information. This work has yet to be presented in a comprehensive manner, nor has it been framed in relation to the current prevailing psychological and scientific models.

For the purposes of this text, medical DMT is defined as the application of DMT services for people with primary medical illness, their caregivers and family members. It also includes the theoretical constructs that inform this specialization and the research approaches that support it. This book reflects the author's perspective that, in the medical realm, DMT functions primarily as a psychosocial support intervention, complementary to conventional and standard medical treatments.

The first challenge in describing a new specialty is to define its boundaries. This task is especially difficult in relation to medical DMT. The medicalization of mental health in the U.S., marked by a shift during the 1980s and 1990s towards more pharmacological intervention and less psychotherapeutic intervention, has blurred the distinction between medical and non-medical disorders. The *Diagnostic and Statistical Manual of Mental Disorders* (4th edition) of the American Psychiatric Association (or APA) (1994) notes that "there is much 'physical' in 'mental' disorders and much 'mental' in 'physical' disorders" and that the distinction is in fact "a reductionistic anachronism of the mind/body dualism" (p.xxi).

However, the following limits have been placed on this book, if only to bring a potentially vast subject into a manageable scope. The book does not cover the treatment of those disorders traditionally identified as primarily psychiatric or behavioral in nature. In the same way, developmental disorders, such as mental retardation, those on the autism–PDD spectrum, and ADD/ADHD, are not included. Despite the obvious and strong neurological component in these conditions, DMT in these areas has been well described elsewhere in the literature and does not represent an emerging specialty within DMT. The book will include review of work in three areas that could be considered in either category:

neurorehabilitation, such as recovery from stroke or traumatic brain injury, work with psychogenic somatic disorders, and medically fragile, seriously neurologically impaired children.

The book is organized into three main parts. Part I provides theoretical and scientific underpinnings to medical DMT. Part II describes examples of work to date in the field, with an emphasis on work by dance/movement therapists in the U.S. The book is by no means exhaustive; there are many dance/movement therapists in the U.S. and abroad providing services to medically involved populations. The material presented in this book is simply representative, and, in this author's judgment, of sound quality. Clinical case examples are incorporated throughout the text, with pseudonyms for all patients and DMT participants.

Part III proposes areas for future development of the specialty with foci on research, education of our colleagues in health care, and professional preparation. Suggestions for clinical tasks and training exercises will be included where appropriate. Sources for the book include published literature, doctoral dissertations, Master's theses, and the author's own experiences providing, researching and teaching medical DMT. The book also includes new material obtained in telephone interviews with medical DMT practitioners from across the U.S. These specialists, Judith R. Bunney, Linni Deihl, Susan Imus, Nicholas Kasovac and Pat Mowry Rutter, generously contributed their time, experience, opinions and wisdom so that this text could include information about their valuable and groundbreaking work. Interviews were conducted in 2002, and are referenced herein as personal communication. Biographies of interviewees can be found in Appendix B.

Foundational concepts for medical dance/movement therapy

This section presents several concepts germane to medical DMT. Together they form the scaffolding of a theoretical foundation for this specialization.

The biopsychosocial model

Engel (1977), in a seminal article that inspired some of the most important research in mind/body medicine, proposed a biopsychosocial model for health care. He envisioned a model that "includes the patient as well as the illness" (p.133) and where the "doctor's task is to account for the dysphoria and the dysfunction which lead individuals to seek medical help, adopt the sick role, and accept the status of patienthood. He must weight the relative contributions of social and psychological as well as of biological factors…" (p.133). Engel argued against what he called the reductionistic, mind–body dualism of the biomedical model, identifying an origin of this thinking in the European Christian church of the fifteenth century. In the years following Engel's publication, there would be a host of leaders and researchers developing and adapting theories toward more wholistic, interdisciplinary health care. DMT and other mental health specialties have benefited from the introduction of the biopsychosocial model into modern medical arenas (Blumenthal, Matthews and Weiss 1993).

Along with the articulation of the biopsychosocial model, the idea of wholism, and the tenets of systems theory have found their way into mainstream health care discussions. Multidisciplinarity and interdisciplinarity are considered essential in any efforts to actualize these ideals in practice. What follows is a brief review of these concepts as might be applicable to the provision of DMT in medical settings.

Tapp and Warner (1985), writing from the perspective of behavioral medicine, considered the philosophy of science and described that worldview as mechanistic and monocausal, concerned with "objectifiable matter-energy and space-time phenomena" (p.6). They observed that behavioral medicine and a multisystems perspective heralded:

> …a partial shift in these basic assumptions to a paradigm that has been labeled "holistic". According to this view, the world is seen from a hierarchical perspective within which matter, energy, space, time, life, and nonlife are transformations within the same ordered unity. The metaphysics of the holistic paradigm is thus monistic, stressing the unity of the phenomena of the universe. For the holistic paradigm, truth is to be found in the interaction between the knower and the external world and involves both inner experience and external verification. (1985, p.6)

Schwartz (1982) drew on Pepper's categories of "world hypotheses" to examine various views of health and illness. They are:

1.   Formistic – binary and categorical, "either–or" thinking.

2.   Mechanistic – single-cause/single-effect thinking, also of an "either–or" nature.

3.   Contextual – an essentially relational style necessary to systems thinking, in which all is multi-caused.

4.   Organistic – interactive, context-sensitive thinking.

Schwartz explains that organistic thinking is "and" thinking in which "combinations of causes are believed to lead to the emergence of new phenomenon and hence, new 'wholes' "(p.1042). It is oriented to patterns, wholistic in nature, and the essence of a systems perspective. According to Schwartz, Western medical science has emphasized a combination of formistic and mechanistic perspectives, but several Eastern approaches have used contextual thinking. The biopsychosocial approach reflects Pepper's second two ways of approaching the world: contextual and organistic. Theoretical contributions in DMT also reflect contextual and organistic perspectives (Kestenberg 1975; Lewis 1979/1994, 2002; Pallaro 1993).

Systems theory

Systems theory is familiar to most mental health professionals because it is the bedrock of family therapy. However, systems theory is a transdisciplinary concept originating with the sciences, particularly physics and biology (von Bertalanffy 1968), and employed in fields as diverse as immunology and computer technology. Systems theory views groups, families, biological, social and individual processes as interacting networks, wholes being more than the sum of parts; each "whole" with active homeostasis (or interaction between equilibrium and disequilibrium); with rules, permeable boundaries and relationships with other systems (Scheflen with Scheflen1972). The concepts have enabled dance/movement therapists to understand, for example, that movement behavior takes on meaning at multiple levels simultaneously (Davis 1990) and that clinical assessment through movement must consider interactional, cultural, developmental, anatomical and psychological aspects (Dulicai 1995). Systems theory undergirds the biopsychosocial model and informs DMT practice in medical contexts. A brief review of the characteristics of systems can highlight how.

Tapp and Warner (1985) outline six properties of systems: wholeness, hierarchical organization, interdependence, self-maintenance, activity and self-transformation. Three of these lead directly to a rationale for dance/movement therapy's role in general health care. First, an understanding of *self-maintenance* equips one for appreciating the physiological dynamics in human health and illness:

> Most control systems operate on the basis of negative feedback. It is to be assumed that within every system there is an internal sensing device whose function is to monitor the state of the internal environment. When deviations occur outside the range of "normal" the control mechanism is initiated. The detector system continues to test the state of the environment and when balance is restored the control mechanism is shut off. (Tapp and Warner 1985, p.9)

Self-transformation refers to:

> the capacity of systems to transform their properties, including their form and structure, over time. Such changes can occur at the same or at higher or lower hierarchical levels. Alterations in the structure of systems thus become an essential component to system survival... Overlapping and alternating feedback loops allow the system to transform itself (i.e., to learn, within any given level of the hierarchy). (Tapp and Warner 1985, p.8)

Third, *activity* is:

> a property of systems that emphasizes the process of transformations that constitute the continual interaction among system elements. Systems are neither static nor reactive. The feedback loops that interrelate system elements insure activity as a constant condition of the system within and between hierarchies. (Tapp and Warner 1985, p.8)

One might consider these properties – self-maintenance (control systems within systems), activity as a constant condition, and a system's capacity for self-transformation – in terms of a distressed or ill individual. It is also possible to conceive of DMT operating on these same principles. The basic DMT techniques of reflecting the patient's movement initiations and guiding the patient through improvisational processes imply a confidence on the therapist's part that something within the patient is going to effect the desired changes. The basic premise that changes occurring on the movement level will generalize to other areas of functioning (Schmais 1974) manifests the systems theory understanding of self-transformation. The notion that human systems are at some level always active provides an avenue for movement intervention regardless of the individual's capacity for overt physical action.

Interdisciplinarity

DMT is an interdisciplinary field: a hybrid of the art of dance and the science of psychology adapted to human service. The field has a history of embracing theories and findings from various other fields including sociology, cultural anthropology, applied kinesiology, traditional healing systems and an assortment of other mind/body approaches. It is not surprising, then, that the field also extends to incorporate the scientific information from medical science, and adapts clinical methods to the needs of medical patients. The challenge of interdisciplinarity is keenly felt in traditional academic contexts where research is conducted. Psychoneuroimmunology (PNI) is one area of research where interdisciplinary bridges have been well built, due in part to attitudes like the one expressed below by Robert Ader, the acknowledged father of PNI.

> PNI is perhaps, the most recent example of an interdisciplinary field that has developed and now prospers by exploring and tilling fertile territories secreted by the arbitrary and illusory boundaries of the biomedical sciences. Disciplinary boundaries and the bureaucracies they spawned are biological fictions that can restrict imagination and the transfer and application of technologies. They lend credence to Werner Heisenberg's assertion that "What we observe is not nature itself, but nature exposed to our method of questioning." Our own language, too, must change. (Ader 1996, p.17)

The clinical arena, with its atmosphere of competition for scarce resources, seems to pose even more of a challenge to true collaboration. Schwartz uses a systems perspective to shed light on the problem:

> The distinction between bodies of knowledge and persons specifically trained in bodies of knowledge is fundamental to understanding a deep implication of system's theory... Hence, what should determine the specific roles that particular person plays in research, education and practice is an interaction of (a) the bodies of knowledge they actually know, (b) the bodies of knowledge necessary to conceptualize and solve the problems comprehensively and (c) legal and ethical principles that theoretically should reflect (a) and (b)... On the research side, the above issues are relatively straightforward. However, on the clinical side (especially in clinical practice *per se*), the recommendations become more controversial and can evoke strong emotions on all sides... No one discipline, by definition, represents all of this information [on biopsychosocial aspects]. What is often confused, however, is that medicine is not a discipline – it is an interdiscipline that primarily operates as a profession. (Schwartz 1982, p.1050)

It is important that dance/movement therapists and their colleagues in other health care specialties find ways to forge new working relationships that will yield creative clinical programming and research. In my view, this is the only way that DMT services can be made available and relevant to people struggling with medical illness. The work related in Part II of this book are examples of successful interdisciplinary efforts.

The mind/body integration

The mind/body connection can be generally defined as the interaction and integration between aspects of human functioning typically considered of the mind and those typically considered of the body. The reciprocal nature of the mind/

body dynamic is a basic premise of DMT (Schmais 1974). Research in this area is discovering that in many ways the distinction between mind and body is arbitrary (Fehder and Douglas 2001; Pert *et al.* 1985). However, to facilitate a review of literature relevant to medical DMT, this book adopts the commonly accepted categorizations. Functions of the mind generally include thinking, communication, intentional behavior, beliefs, attitudes, relationships, social processes and expression of emotions. Functions of the body encompass physiologic, kinesiologic, neurologic, hormonal and immunologic systems.

The phenomenon is widely accepted in popular culture and researched from almost every imaginable academic angle. Scholars in philosophy, religion, ethics, anthropology, history, the arts, the basic sciences and the behavioral sciences have investigated the mind/body connection using the particular research methods of their respective disciplines (Klivington 1997; Moyers 1993; Yardley 1996). The body of knowledge has grown exponentially in the last two decades, and a comprehensive review is beyond the scope of this book. (For an overview of the clinical science research on the topic, see Dienstfrey 2001.) The work to be reviewed in this volume focuses only on theory and research that specifically inform the practice of DMT with primarily medically ill patients and their loved ones. Chapter 3 is devoted to a review of relevant scientific findings.

The U.S. National Institutes of Health (NIH) have categorized DMT as a mind/body intervention, and in a report to the NIH by several experts in complementary and alternative medicine (CAM) (Achterberg *et al.* 1994) these approaches were introduced as follows:

> In approaching the field of mind–body interventions, it is important that the mind not be viewed as if it were dualistically isolated from the body, as if it were doing something to the body. Mind–body relations are always mutual and bi-directional – the body affects the mind and is affected by it. [...]When the term mind–body is used in this report, therefore, there is no implication that an object or thing – the mind – is somehow acting on a separate entity – the body. Rather, "mind–body" could perhaps best be regarded as an overall process that is not easily dissected into separate and distinct components or parts. (Achterberg *et al.* 1994, p.4)

Rossi (1993), integrates work in neuroscience and physics (see Klivington 1997) and approaches the process in terms of information:

> Mind and body are not separate phenomena, one being somehow spirit and the other matter. Mind and body are both aspects of one information system. Life is an information system. Biology is a process of information

transduction. Mind and body are two facets or two ways of conceptualizing this single information system. (p.67)

The reader will easily recognize in these descriptions two central aspects of DMT: the reciprocal or bidirectional influences of mind and body and the notion that their relationship is a process. In the chapters to follow, various other aspects of the mind/body interaction will be discussed.

Quality of life

Quality of life is gaining attention in psychology and behavioral medicine as a relevant health outcome and worthy of clinical focus. The definition of *quality of life* is not yet clearly operationalized for mental health populations (Gladis *et al.* 1999), but several overarching components have been identified. These include "functional status (what one is capable of doing), access to resources, opportunities to use one's abilities to pursue interests and a sense of well-being" (Lehman 1999, p.175).

Health related quality of life (HRQOL) is a construct pertaining specifically to those living with a primary medical illness. The HRQOL framework emphasizes, "the specific impacts that disease, injury, and their prevention and treatment have on the value of survival" (Lehman 1999, p.175). There are many ways to assess quality of life, including several disease-specific assessment instruments. Most rely on self-report, based on the understanding that it is the patient's own perceptions of his or her life that are most relevant. Dimensions of HRQOL include physical functioning, role limitations caused by physical health problems, role limitations caused by emotional problems, social functioning, emotional well-being, energy/ fatigue, pain, and general health perceptions (Hays and Morales 2001). Patients seem to distinguish between quality of life and actual health status, with the former being more associated with mental health than with physical functioning (Smith, Avis and Assmann 1999). One implication of this finding is that interventions designed to enhance mental health may bring about as much or more quality of life improvement than medical treatment aimed solely at physical functioning. Jankey (1999) studied 100 long-term hospital care patients and learned that for them, meaningfulness in life was the strongest predictor of quality of life. The variables of optimism, a sense of control, perception of one's disability, understanding on one's illness, satisfaction with social support, personal accomplishments, and future goals were also associated with better quality of life.

It is possible to view the potential impact of DMT and other psychosocial or mind/body approaches from a quality of life standpoint, especially for the medically ill. DMT often focuses on goals such as the enhancement of emotional well-being, meaningfulness, optimism, goal setting, the sense of control, self-perception and social functioning. Loughlin's (1993) report of work with teens and women who have Turner's Syndrome is an example. Struggling with abnormally short stature and pubertal development, these women practiced using forceful movement and making clearly formed shapes in space during their DMT sessions. Some of the participants were soon making proactive changes in their lives such as leaving unsatisfactory jobs and reporting more assertiveness in relationships. The participants themselves credited DMT with empowering them to become less passive in their own lives.

The value of any intervention that can positively impact self-perceived quality of life should not be understated. Sobel (1995) considers psychosocial interventions for their cost effectiveness, noting that:

> Patients' psychosocial and medical needs are addressed through stress management techniques, psychoeducation, psychotherapy, and emotional support... Rather than targeting specific diseases, these psychosocial interventions may operate by influencing underlying, shared determinants of health... Variously termed hardiness, optimism, self-efficacy, sense of coherence, sense of control, sense of connectedness, happiness and pleasure, the core factors are related to a wide range of [positive health] outcomes. (p.237)

With quality of life as an overarching goal of medical DMT, the distinctions between curing and healing, and between illness and disease become important.

Disease/illness

If mainstream health care is to routinely include psychosocial as well as biomedical interventions, the separate contributions of each need to be defined and appreciated. Achterberg (1985) credited the behavioral and social sciences with making relevant the distinction between illness and disease. She characterizes illness as the "unique personal impact of mental or physical pathology" and disease as "the pathology itself" (p.9). Kleinman detailed this further: "Let us call disease any primary malfunctioning in biological and psychological processes. And let us call illness the secondary psychosocial and cultural responses to disease, e.g., how the patient, his family, and social network react to his disease" (Kleinman 1973, as cited in Achterberg 1985, p.145).

Using the definitions above, it is suggested that as with other forms of psychosocial support, DMT addresses the illness, but not the disease.

Curing/healing

Once the differences between disease and illness are understood and adopted, the parallel distinctions between curing and healing come to the fore. Achterberg and others (1994) proposed that curing is the actual eradication of a disease, while healing implies a sense of wholeness and completeness (p.4). Feeling better, or more whole, can be an outcome of healing and attending to the illness rather than the disease. Kleinman and Sung (1979, as cited in Achterberg 1985) observed that the term "healing" is awkward in conventional health care circles, but that we need to keep in mind the often separate perspectives of patients and their physicians. They state that "patients and physicians maintain two separate sets of criteria with which they judge medical outcome, with physicians tending to identify biological change, and patients opting for the more subjective component of 'feeling better,' as the appropriate variables" (p.145).

Kaplan (1990) argued that real health outcome is always behavioral, because it is the patient's ability to function and live life as he or she envisions it that is the critical measure of health status. These subjective assessments of the patient's own experience are as meaningful as any biological indicator of disease processes. After life expectancy, quality of life and the ability to function are the most important criteria in health assessment and treatment outcome, according to Kaplan. This view is especially pertinent in chronic conditions, when the patient learns to live with disease, and the enhancement or maintenance of function and meaning are primary concerns.

Patients reinforce this distinction every day. In a study of DMT for adults with cystic fibrosis, a chronic and usually fatal disease (Goodill 1995), I described the brief treatment to a new participant. His face lit up with recognition and he said, "Sure, I get it. Since there's no cure, we may as well work on healing." Another patient in that study told his nurse about the DMT session he had just experienced and how he enjoyed the relaxation with guided imagery portion. He exclaimed, "She cured my CF!" While confusing the definitions of curing and healing that are presented above, this young man illustrated Kleinman's point perfectly: for patients, simply feeling better can be the most important outcome.

The context of medical dance/movement therapy

This section will position medical DMT in the context of related disciplines such as complementary and alternative medicine, mind/body medicine, arts medicine, dance medicine, dance and health or health benefits of dancing, behavioral medicine, exercise physiology, and the other creative arts therapies (i.e., medical art therapy, medical music therapy, music medicine, drama and poetry).

Complementary and alternative medicine

Complementary and alternative medicine (CAM) encompasses a vast range of disciplines and is defined by the U.S. National Institutes of Health's (NIH) National Center for Complementary and Alternative Medicine (NCCAM) in an exclusionary fashion as "a group of diverse medical and health care systems, practices, and products that are not presently considered to be part of conventional medicine" (National Institutes of Health n.d.). CAM therapies are typically wholistic, many are preventative in nature, and some derive from cultural worldviews inconsistent with the values manifest in mainstream biomedical systems. The NIH Office of Alternative Medicine (now the NCCAM) was established in 1993 as the nation's official clearing house and funder of CAM research. The agency currently delineates five categories of therapies, including:

- alternative medical systems
- biologically based therapies
- energy therapies
- manipulative and body-based methods, and
- mind/body interventions.

As mentioned above, DMT is included in the last category which is described by the NIH as follows: "Mind–body interventions employ a variety of techniques designed to facilitate the mind's capacity to affect bodily functions and symptoms" (National Institutes of Health n.d.). It is apparent that not all branches of CAM actively and intentionally involve the mind/body interactions, and even the NIH definition implies a unidirectional dynamic (mind influencing body), with the desired change in the physical realm. Also included in NIH's mind/body intervention category are the other creative arts therapies, hypnosis, and imagery based techniques. Micozzi (1997) has commented that the creative arts therapies typify the problem in CAM that there is not easy access to enough practitioners to bring the services to the mainstream.

Massage therapy is included in the NIH's category of manipulative and body-based methods and therapeutic touch is included as an energy therapy. Both differ from DMT in that the patient is generally passive and receptive to the ministrations of the practitioner. Like DMT, these therapies both involve a conscious exchange of energy between patient and practitioner, and both rely on the bidirectional dynamic of the mind/body integration. Therapeutic touch is described as "an intentionally directed process of energy modulation during which the practitioner uses the hands as a focus to assess and mobilize the healee's energy field, with compassionate intention…" (Ireland and Olson 2000, p.57).

Therapeutic touch is slightly controversial in mainstream medical circles, and research on its efficacy is ongoing (Winstead-Fry and Kijek 1999). Researchers of massage therapy have repeatedly demonstrated its benefits to both psychological and physical health. Some of these findings will be presented in subsequent chapters.

Mind/body medicine

Mind/body medicine is a closely related area, as evidenced by the definitions excerpted below. The first is from Deepak Chopra, M.D., a well-known proponent and leader of the field:

> The essential foundation of mind/body medicine is the recognition that for every experience in the mind, there is a corresponding change in the physiology and biochemistry of our body. We have a vast internal pharmacy that can be accessed through conscious choices we make in our lives. A key tenet of mind/body medicine is that health is not the mere absence of disease. Rather, it is the dynamic integration of our environment, body, mind and spirit. (Chopra n.d.)

At Harvard University's Center for Mind/Body Medicine, founded by Herbert Benson, M.D., the terms *mind/body medicine* and *behavioral medicine* are used interchangeably, and a "mind/body/spirit model of care" is employed with a multifactorial and wholistic approach. Spiritual well-being is described as belief that one's life has meaning and purpose. For the team at Harvard, "The mind/body/spirit relationship implies that if you address only one of these factors you may not be able to achieve the best possible results" (Center for Mind/Body Medicine 1999). CAM methods used in the center emphasize yoga, meditation and the elicitation of the relaxation response (Benson 1975). It has been suggested that the growth of mind/body medicine practices may actually signal the return of psychology into the practice of medicine (Taylor 2000).

The field of mind/body medicine has made important scientific progress explaining and harnessing the potentials of the mind/body interaction. Examples include the work of Ernest Rossi and others with clinical hypnosis, and that of Jeanne Achterberg and colleagues with imagery.

Creative arts therapies

Other creative arts therapies, notably art therapy and music therapy, have established a strong base of expertise and research in medical applications (Loewy 1997; Malchiodi 1993, 1999a, 1999b). The field of music therapy has made strides in tracking health beneficial physiological responses to music and music therapy interventions across a wide range of populations (Bittman *et al.* 2001; Burns *et al.* 2001; Coleman *et al.* 1998). Guided Imagery and Music™ has shown benefits for a variety of medical populations, including quality of life and mood state improvement in cancer patients (Jacobi 1995; Summer 1990). Creativity as a process and a trait has much to offer the practice of medicine (Dossey 2001; Rodenhauser 1996). Rodenhauser stated:

> creativity from both internal and external sources has deeply personal – and spiritual – implications. It provides affirmation, passion, expression, excitement, and experience of a universal nature. It provides the means to modify reality, to make the ordinary extraordinary, and to advance knowledge and culture. Along with humanism in medicine, it ranks among the highest forms of giving. (p.6)

He recommended creative activity to health care professionals as a way of enhancing their ability to keep a human perspective in their work. Dossey suggested that play and creativity will cultivate the typically undervalued traits of empathy, altruism and compassion in health care professionals.

Arts medicine

Another related emerging field is arts medicine. It has a close relationship to the arts therapies and to other practices in the mind/body intervention arena. Arts medicine is concerned with the various interrelationships between the arts and health care. These include: the artistic lives of health care providers, the history of medicine through the study of arts, the esthetics of health care environments, works of art by people living with disease and arts-based services to patients and their families (largely, the creative arts therapies). The International Arts Medicine Association (IAMA) names, as one of its eight goals, "to promote the creative arts therapy movement, which studies the healing potential of the arts for individuals, institutions and society" (IAMA 2001). Richard Lippin, M.D., a poet and the founder of IAMA, states that he has "caught glimpses of the promised land in Arts-Medicine but only by standing on the shoulders of the leaders of the creative arts therapy movement…" (Lippin 1997). Widespread interest in arts medicine spawned the refereed journal, the *International Journal of Arts Medicine*, which contains work by many creative arts therapists.

Arts medicine is an inclusive and growing field, open to new discoveries and new types of practitioners. Among the handful of successful arts medicine programs in the U.S., the Artists-in-Residence program and the Center for the Arts in Healthcare Research and Education at Shands Hospital in Gainesville, Florida, are notable for the creative, robust nature of their vision and actualization (Graham-Pole and Lane 1994). The renowned physician and clown Patch Adams, M.D., is affiliated with the arts medicine movement, as it embodies this part of his philosophy of health care: "Art is not an indulgence, secondary to medical activities, but is fundamental to the practice of interdisciplinary medicine" (Adams and Mylander 1993, p.86). Adams is referring to art in the sense of all the arts, including dance. He espouses the health benefits of humor and fun as well, and this claim is upheld by a number of research studies (Burns 1996; Cogan, Cogan-Waltz and McCue 1987, as cited in Salovey *et al.* 2000).

Health psychology

Health psychology was formalized as a specialty division of the American Psychological Association (Division 38) in 1978. Health psychology "seeks to advance contributions of psychology to the understanding of health and illness through basic and clinical research, education, and service activities and encourages the integration of biomedical information about health and illness with current psychological knowledge" (American Psychological Association n.d.). Health psychology is considered a subset of behavioral medicine and is a critical source of theory and research information for dance/movement therapists who work with medical populations. The field provides "theoretical and conceptual frameworks that elucidate the (non)practice of health behaviors, the role of stress in affecting illness and illness behavior, the representations that people hold regarding their health and illness and the determinants of their adjustment to it" (Taylor 1990). Recently, the field has studied optimism and motivation from the positive psychology framework as well (Folkman and Moskowitz 2000). Much of Chapter 2 is devoted to material generated by health psychologists and their collaborators.

Dance and movement

Another context of DMT is in relation to other dance and movement forms. Dancing alone seems to provide certain health benefits (Hanna 1988, 1995), including the reduction of anxiety (Leste and Rust 1984). Dance as community expression and ritual has been examined by Hanna (1988), who explains the physiological processes induced in traditional dance healing rituals. Graduate projects by Halperin (1995) and Watson (2001) are examples of research exploring the similarities between dance healing rituals and DMT. Dance healing rituals constitute an ancient and global rationale for the exploration of dance services such as DMT in modern health care. Movement disciplines such as yoga and Qi-gong have also been investigated by CAM researchers (Singh *et al.* 1998).

As DMT takes its place in the general health care system among the array of mind/body modalities and creative/expressive approaches, it is useful to identify the intrinsic and unique features of DMT that make it a suitable treatment option for medically involved patients. Melsom (1999) considered the suitability of DMT with medical populations, and articulated five intrinsic features of DMT as follows:

- the integration of mind, body, emotions, creativity and spirituality
- the inclusion of relaxation, breathwork and imagery within the therapeutic process
- the use of touch, mirroring, synchrony and body empathy
- the facilitation of work towards new ways of physical and emotional coping
- the promotion of emotional healing (p.175).

She further identified four characteristics of DMT that distinguish it from other psychosocial support interventions in typical biomedical health care settings:

- the incorporation of the body into the psychotherapeutic process
- the building of a relationship with the patient's body
- the promotion of the establishment or re-establishment of a positive relationship between the patient and his or her body, and
- the use of creative movement expression to promote the expression of health (p.170).

In addition to these, DMT differs from several other mind/body disciplines in that in DMT, the patient's own expressive initiations become the content of the session, and unfold in an interactive and improvisational manner. Usually, the dance/movement therapist follows the patient into whatever themes or issues emerge as most salient. This is in contrast to the practitioner-led and often routine sequences used in movement disciplines like yoga, Qi-gong or tai chi. The active nature of the patient's participation in DMT is likewise in contrast to the more passive patient experience in treatment modalities like therapeutic touch or massage therapy. Like many other CAM, mind/body and psychotherapeutic approaches with medically ill patients, DMT and the other creative arts therapies employ imagery. However, Gorelick (1989) noted that the creative arts therapies are unique in the psychotherapeutic world because of their reliance on imagery, symbol and metaphor as a central mechanism of the therapy. Taking these notions together, five core foci for medical DMT are proposed:

- vitality
- coping (primarily relationship-focused coping)
- self-efficacy
- body image of illness
- mood.

These features of and foci for medical DMT will reappear in the DMT clinical work that is described in the chapters to follow.

CHAPTER 2

Psychological Concepts for Medical Dance/Movement Therapy

There is ample evidence for the premise that in the treatment of medical illnesses, psychosocial factors must be addressed. First, comorbidity of physical and psychiatric illness is substantial. Sobel (1995) reports that "although 10%–20% of patients presenting in a primary care setting have a diagnosable psychiatric disorder, more than 80% have evidence of significant psychological distress" (p.235). Depression is of particular concern with estimates that 10–14 per cent of people in medical inpatient units are depressed (Brody 1998). The prevalence of medical illness among cases of completed suicide ranges from 30–40 per cent, with the greatest risk among patients with HIV/AIDS, multiple sclerosis and brain cancers (Hughes and Kleespies 2001).

In addition to the obvious benefits of reducing depression and the risk of suicide, there can be cost savings in the health care system when psychosocial issues are addressed. One review of cost offset data (Friedman *et al.* 1995) delineates six different pathways through which psychological, social or educational interventions reduce utilization of conventional medical resources and produce cost savings. These savings have been achieved with conditions as diverse as childhood fever, arthritis, tobacco addiction and post-surgical complications.

Chapter 1 identified health psychology and behavioral medicine research as significant sources of knowledge to inform medical dance/movement therapy (DMT) and other psychosocial support modalities. Here, a number of key constructs will be reviewed, selected for the particular ways that these concepts and phenomena may relate to the premises and practice of medical DMT. Quality of life, stress, coping, self-efficacy and adherence, social support, emotions and affect, positive psychology, spirituality, imagery, and altered states will all be discussed in the pages to follow. The discussion is limited to a rather cursory overview of each. The interested reader is encouraged to pursue the extensive research literature that is devoted to every one of these themes. For comprehensive coverage of these and related topics, the reader is also referred to a recent volume by Battino (2001). Each concept is presented under its own subheading, defined and described using theory and research literature. Examples of related interventions, those with potential relevance for the practice of medical DMT, will be given with research findings when available. There are multiple overlaps between these elements of mind/body health, yet the question of how these factors influence health is pertinent to all.

Theorists have developed several models for explaining the mechanisms by which such factors such as stress threaten health. For example, self-efficacy and social support provide a "buffering" effect against disease (Cohen 1997). The *direct and indirect effects* model, as presented by Smith and Nicassio (1995), has bearing here. They state, "psychosocial factors may have direct, indirect or moderating influences on health outcomes" (p.9). Direct effects are relationships that "do not require mediation by other processes and, in essence, describe a closed loop" between the factor and the health outcome (p.9). An example is the relationship between anxiety and muscle tension. Indirect pathways of influence may operate when (in the case of threats to health) social isolation leads to poor adherence to self-care regimens and thus to a decline in health status. Positive indirect effects of social support may, for example, lead to smoking cessation, which may enhance health. If a factor is an essential ingredient in a health outcome, it is known as a *mediator* of that effect. When a factor plays a role in the course of a disease, but does not explain it entirely, it is known as a *moderator* of the health effect (Smith and Nicassio, p.10). Cohen (1988) observed that there are several possible points of entry in the pathways linking psychosocial factors and disease/health status. Sobel (1995) imagined "disease superhighways" (p.234), a common set of psychophysiological processes through which psychosocial and environment risk factors exert their influence on health, possibly by altering the individual's susceptibility to infection and disease. One such process is the familiar "fight–flight" or stress response (Cannon 1932; Selye 1956/1976) that stimulates the production of hormones and other substances to weaken the immune system, leaving the individual more susceptible to disease. On the other hand, the "relaxation response" (Benson 1975) activates the parasympathetic nervous system, leading to hormone release thought to be health enhancing. These and other psychophysiological processes will be discussed further in Chapter 3.

As of this writing, mechanisms by which DMT may bring about positive changes in overall health have been explored (e.g., Krantz 1994) but not clearly identified. Nonetheless, the literature reviewed here leads to a presumption that indirect effects play a role. For example, if poor body awareness renders a patient unable to report levels of pain accurately, physicians will not be able to prescribe appropriate pain medication. If DMT can increase body awareness, leading to better pain reporting, it will be influencing the pain at an indirect level.

The placebo effect is another mind/body phenomenon that has generated interest in both the CAM and mainstream medical communities (Achterberg *et al.* 1994; NIH 2001). It is a controversial occurrence that has been defined as "desirable physiological or psychological effects attributable to the use of inert medications" (NIH 2001, p.1) and which has implications for clinical trials research as well as clinical practice. Those who study the placebo effect from a mind/body perspective focus on it as "a change in a patient's illness attributable to the symbolic import of a treatment rather than a specific pharmacologic or physiological property" (Turner *et al.* 1994, p.1610). Rossi (1993) describes the response broadly as a "general, automatic mind–body communication that utilizes physical treatment methods to reduce anxiety and facilitate healing by marshalling powerful cultural expectations and beliefs in the treatment method" (p.18). Norman Cousins has famously called the placebo effect "the doctor within" (Cousins 1979, p.69, as cited in Rossi 1993, p.14). The placebo effect is fairly common, by some estimates accounting for up to 30 per cent of medical improvement (Achterberg *et al.* 1994). As reflected in Rossi's definition, researchers have begun to "unpack" the mystery of the placebo response by investigating its various components. They include the patient's beliefs about and expectations for the treatment, the presence of a suggestion (generally from the clinician) that the treatment will work, the quality of the patient–provider relationship, and a decrease in the patient's anxiety. As these components have been identified, there has been a suggestion that we no longer use the term *placebo*, which relegates these powerful factors to the accidental and the peripheral, but instead adopt the term *non-specific effects* (Turner *et al.* 1994). This is where psychosocial factors and interventions may come in. It has been suggested that the placebo or non-specific effect "must be considered as an important component...of all behavioral interventions" (Hall, Anderson and O'Grady 1994, p.192). Others maintain that non-specific effects become quite specific when understood (Moerman and Jonas 2002) and consider instead the *meaning response*. The meaning response is "the physiologic or psychological effects of meaning in the origins or treatment of illness" (Moerman and Jonas 2002, p.472). If spontaneous healing has to do with factors such as meaning, beliefs and relationship, psychosocial concerns and mind/body dynamics should logically assume a central role in multidisciplinary health care.

As outlined in Chapter 1, in the context of primary medical illness, DMT and other psychosocial interventions primarily address quality of life issues. In the field at large, quality of life is described and measured with both objective criteria (e.g., functioning in daily activities, or ability to return to work, etc.) and by the more subjective perceptions of the patient him/herself. This book emphasizes the second approach, with the patient's perceptions in the foreground, to guide discussion of other concepts and to inform treatment.

Stress

A stressor is an event, a physical or psychological threat or trauma, that occurs outside the individual. Stress is the individual's response to that threat, and depends on the way the stressor is perceived, or appraised. Shock, grief and fear are all manifestations of the stress response. Stress is considered a "negative emotional experience accompanied by predictable biochemical, physiological, and behavioral changes that are directed toward adaptation either by manipulating the situation to alter the stressor or by accommodating its effects" (Baum 1990, p.653). It is a "whole body phenomenon" (Baum 1990, p.658). The transactional perspective of stress emphasizes the interface between the person and his or her environment. In this framework, stress occurs when there is "some form of imbalance between the demands imposed upon an individual and the resources available to accommodate" (Monroe 1989, p.513) or, simply put, when demands outstrip resources. Thus, two people may experience the same event quite differently as a function of the resources they each bring to the situation and how they each appraise it. In this appraisal, "individuals evaluate the significance of an event for their well-being and their ability to rally resources to manage its demands" (Lobel and Dunkel-Schetter 1990, p.215). The event itself may be positive or negative, but a stress response to it is almost always a negative one. The characteristics of events that contribute to their potential to induce stress, include intensity, immediacy and the degree of danger or harm involved (Baum 1990). Individual characteristics that seem to moderate the stress response include:

1.   habituation to similar situations (Lobel and Dunkel-Schetter 1990)

2.   the presence of social supports, and

3.   the types of coping employed (see below).

Chronic stress is a related but unique problem in that it may outlast the existence of the initial stressor itself (Baum 1990). In terms of health status, it is a risk factor that exacerbates conditions across the entire disease continuum. Caregivers of the seriously or chronically medically ill, including spouses of coronary heart disease patients (Coyne 2000), family members of cancer patients (Fawzy and Fawzy

1994) and bereaved partners of those with AIDS (Taylor *et al.* 2000) are at measurable health risk, ostensibly due to the unremitting demands placed upon them. Chronic inadequate resources make those who live in poverty particularly vulnerable to the everyday stressors of their environment (Watts-Jones 1990). As mentioned above, the stress response and chronic stress form one possible common disease pathway in the link between psychological, emotional and biological processes.

Many mind/body medicine programs provide stress reduction interventions. Good results have been obtained in studies of mindfulness-based meditation (Reibel *et al.* 2001), and other methods that induce the relaxation response (Hall and O'Grady 1991; Kutz, Borsyenko and Benson 1985). Among health care workers, interventions involving massage, music relaxation with visual imagery, muscle relaxation and social support have all been effective in reducing stress-related mood variables (Field *et al.* 1997). Hanna (1988) discussed dance as a way to reduce stress and offered this physiological hypothesis for the effect, beginning with the stress response as described by Cannon (1932). She states that "when a person neither fights nor flees because physical action in the immediate situation is inappropriate, biochemical elements of energy may remain in the body" (Hanna 1988, p.11) and the physical activity of dance permits a natural release of stress related hormones. Further, she observed:

> the exercise of dance increases the circulation of blood carrying oxygen to the muscles and the brain and alters the level of certain brain chemicals, as in the stress response pattern. Vigorous dancing induces the release of endorphins thought to produce analgesia and euphoria. (p.12)

These stress reducing benefits of dance, as described by Hanna, are the same as with any type of repetitive, rhythmic, sustained form of exercise, an effect that is well documented (Sherwood 1997).

Coping

Coping may be the most studied psychological phenomenon of the last two decades (Somerfield and McCrae 2000). Coping has been defined as:

> the process of managing external or internal demands that are perceived as taxing or exceeding a person's resources (Lazarus and Folkman 1984). Coping may consist of behaviors and intrapsychic responses designed to overcome, reduce, or tolerate these demands (Lazarus and Launeir 1978). (Taylor 1990, p.44)

Historically, the theory of coping strategies has its roots in psychoanalytic thinking, beginning with Sigmund Freud's descriptions of defense mechanisms and developed further by Anna Freud (1979, originally published 1936). Somerfield and McCrae (2000) are among the contemporary researchers who have appreciated this link, and the possibility that not all coping is necessarily conscious and volitional. Vaillant (2000) discusses the adaptive value of the mature (and often involuntary) defenses including anticipation, suppression, altruism, humor and sublimation. This more expansive thinking bodes well for the mainstreaming of interventions, such as DMT, that emphasize the intuitive, non-verbal, preconscious (Kubie 1958), symbolic and sensed aspects of experience.

In research on psychosocial interventions for cancer patients, Fawzy and Fawzy employ Weisman, Worden and Sobel's work that identified four key ingredients of good coping. They are:

1.   optimism (the expectation of positive change)

2.   practicality (learning that options and alternatives are seldom completely exhausted)

3.   flexibility (changing strategies to reflect the changing nature of the perceived problems)

4.   resourcefulness (Weisman, Worden and Sobel 1980, as cited in Fawzy and Fawzy 1994, p.370).

Coping strategies have been categorized in several different ways. First, *emotion-focused coping* is aimed at reducing or managing the emotional distress while *problem-focused coping* is aimed at problem solving or doing something to alter the source of the stress (Carver, Scheier and Weintraub 1989). People use both: they are interdependent and supplement each other in the process of responding to taxing demands (Lazarus 2000), and there are distinct individual differences or styles for coping. Generally, *active-behavioral coping*, "trying to improve some aspect of the illness by active means such as exercise, use of relaxation techniques, and frequent collaborative consultations with the physician", and *active-cognitive coping* in which "one tries to understand illness and accept [its] ...effect on life by focusing on positive rather than negative changes..." have better health outcomes than do more avoidant methods of coping (Fawzy and Fawzy 1994, p.371).

In the development of a widely used coping assessment scale called COPE, Carver *et al.* (1989) identified 13 dimensions of coping. Because conceptually they have useful clinical implications, the authors' definitions are paraphrased here. *Active coping* is the process of taking active steps to try to remove or circumvent the stressor or to ameliorate its effects. *Planning* is the process of thinking about how to cope with a stressor. *Positive reinterpretation* (or *appraisal*) *and growth* involves the conscious management of one's distress reactions and emotions (see also Folkman and Moskowitz 2000). *Suppression of competing activities* is the act of putting other events and concerns to the side in order to deal with the stressor. *Restraint coping* is holding oneself back and not acting prematurely. The *seeking of social support for emotional reasons* is for getting moral support, understanding or sympathy, and the *seeking of social support for instrumental reasons* is for getting information, advice or assistance. People under stress sometimes *turn to religion* (a factor discussed in more detail below). *Acceptance* is an important coping device when the stressor is something to which the individual must accommodate (rather than change the stressor itself). Two devices are notably maladaptive ways of coping. They include *behavioral disengagement*, which is to reduce one's efforts or even give up in relation to the stressor, and *mental disengagement*, which is to allow oneself to be distracted from thinking about the stressor or dealing with it. The authors posit that *focusing on and venting emotions* is considered sometimes adaptive, as in a period of mourning. However, as a prolonged or sole response emotional venting is generally not congruent with effective coping (Carver *et al.* 1989, pp.268–70). Reviewing evidence for a direct path between coping and health, Billings *et al.* (2000) concluded that "an active, engaged form of coping is associated with better health prognosis, whereas passive, avoidant coping strategies are associated with worse prognosis" (Billings *et al.* 2000, para. 13). Good coping may involve different combinations of strategies for different people at different stages of an illness; it is highly individual and context-dependent.

Denial can be defined as "refusal to believe that the stressor exists or…trying to act as though the stressor is not real" (Carver *et al.* 1989, p.270). Denial is a complex coping phenomenon that is paradoxical. It may be helpful immediately after diagnosis of a life-threatening illness because it enables people to move past the initial and paralyzing fears to mobilize other important coping resources. Sobel (1995) notes, "even people with objective disease seem to do better when they believe themselves to be healthy" (p.236). Some studies have found that the use of denial can predict more rapid medical stabilization in the initial hours and days following a heart attack. However, others show that denial can be associated with declines in psychosocial functioning and compliance following discharge from the hospital (Smith and Nicassio 1995, p.24). Denial may constitute a buffer against the emotionally paralyzing and health-threatening effects of overwhelming anxiety about one's health or life, but when it persists and interferes with adherence to self-care regimens or other forms of active coping, denial is clearly maladaptive.

DMT techniques emphasize awareness of bodily sensations and the emotions that arise from increased sensitivity to one's bodily cues. It would behoove dance/movement therapists and others who use experiential methods to stay aware of this paradox about denial when working with the medically ill. At times, denial is best left intact. The medically ill seem to persist (and sometimes thrive) by maintaining a fragile, yet important balance of emotional self-awareness and other adaptive coping devices (Taylor *et al.* 2000). Respectful attention to the patient's individual constellation of coping strategies and the other stressors impacting life and health is advised. Practically speaking, this may mean sometimes limiting the use of techniques that deepen sensation or uncover less conscious material, so that the patient can titrate the intensity of his or her own emotional experience.

The concept of coping is consistent with the tenets and methods of cognitive behavioral therapy (CBT), which is widely used in the field of behavioral medicine. Interventions are geared towards the recognition of thoughts and assumptions, understanding their impact on symptoms, and problem solving (Massie, Holland and Straker 1989). CBT is usually short term, aimed at control of target symptoms, and often involves homework.

Self-efficacy

Self-efficacy is defined as "the belief that one can successfully perform behaviors to produce a desired outcome" (Berkman 1995, p.251). In health care, this is an important attribute because it leads to better self-care, and as Sobel (1995) points out "self-care is 80% of health care" (p.237). Self-efficacy is a judgment or conviction about oneself; it is the opposite of helplessness. As with quality of life, the patient's perception of his or her own capacities is the key to assessing self-efficacy. According to Berkman, self-efficacy is "shaped by past and present behaviors and by the social environment through observation of behaviors in others and verbal support and persuasion" (p.251). Thus, even if self-efficacy is low at the point of diagnosis, it can be bolstered through interactive and social processes, particularly interventions that encourage independent activity on one's own behalf. As a psychological construct, self-efficacy is related to "health locus of control" (see below) and impacts health outcomes through the behavioral pathways such as adherence. There also may be physiological pathways through which attributes such as self-efficacy exert their influence. Upon reviewing the scientific evidence for this, Sobel claimed, "There is a biology of self-confidence" (1995, p.237). In this statement, he is referring to a cluster of traits that contribute to health, such as optimism, self-efficacy, hardiness and a sense of control.

Health locus of control is an assessment of how much control a person feels over his or her health and the course of an illness. Internal locus of control indicates a sense of responsibility for one's health (Gallagher *et al.* 1989, p.59). Gallagher and colleagues (1989) studied low back pain patients who were unemployed due to their condition. Using a logistic regression analysis and controlling for age and length of time out of work, they found that health locus of control and other psychosocial factors predicted subjects' likelihood of returning to work within six months better than physical or biomechanical factors did.

The term *adherence* refers to a "collaborative involvement of the patient in a mutually acceptable course of behavior that produces a desired preventive or therapeutic result" (Turk and Meichenbaum 1988, p.251). Adherence involves the adoption of good health behaviors. In recent years, the field has replaced the concept of *compliance,* which is a more passive, obedient following of instructions, with adherence. Meaning "to stick together", adherence suggests a partnership and a more active, voluntary process for the patient. Effective communication between provider and patient contributes to adherence, which is critical to good self-care. The relationship between self-efficacy and adherence is complicated by findings that for some chronic disease patients, up to 73 per cent of non-adherence is intentional (Turk and Meichenbaum 1988). The authors surmise that when there is little symptom relief yielded by a demanding, inconvenient and discomforting care regimen, the patient sometimes makes an informed choice not to do it. This is connected to having a sense of control over the disorder and (in chronic conditions) one's life. Curiously, this kind of selective non-adherence is a strategy that can be adaptive when it is flexible and sensitive to day to day fluctuations in disease status (Turk and Meichenbaum 1988 p.259).

In an overview of the field of health psychology, Taylor (1990) summarizes the knowledge about self-care as follows:

> Specifically, we now know that people are most likely to practice a good health measure when (a) the threat to health is severe; (b) the perceived personal vulnerability and/or the likelihood of developing the disorder is high; (c) the person believes that he or she is able to perform the response that will reduce the threat (self-efficacy); and (d) the response is effective in overcoming the threat (response efficacy). (p.41)

Compared to other mind/body disciplines in use throughout the health care system, DMT may be uniquely suited to the goal of increasing self-efficacy and internal health locus of control for medical patients who need intervention in these areas. Unlike methods such as meditation, music-assisted guided imagery or visualization techniques, DMT mobilizes the patient to physical activity in the session. This recalls one component of self-efficacy: activity. Unlike other movement-oriented healing methods such as yoga, Qi-gong or aerobic exercise, the DMT patient usually initiates expressive movement themes. The therapist then guides and shapes those expressions in an improvisational manner. In DMT, rather than being told what to do, the patient has the experience of taking the lead. These features of DMT, patient-initiated physical activity and responsive attention between the therapist and patient to the patient's own perceptions of bodily sensations, combine to replicate the conditions needed for encouraging self-efficacy.

Social support

Social support is a broad term that encompasses social networks, social supports and social relationships. Social support is provided by those with intimate ties such as a spouse, close friends and family, as well as through larger networks such as worship communities, co-worker groups and groups created specifically to provide support. Perceived social support is a relatively stable sense of the "availability of interpersonal resources or integration in a large social network, and is associated with more positive well-being" (Billings et al. 2000, para. 6). Social support and perceived social support have been found to have a stress-buffering effect for those with medical illness (Cohen 1988) and it is through the moderation of stress's impact that social support is believed to influence health status (Monroe 1989). In addition, social support encourages the adoption of positive health behaviors (such as exercising, improving one's diet and taking prescribed medications) and the cessation or reduction of health risky behaviors (such as smoking and excessive alcohol use) (Cohen 1988). The impact of social support is appreciable, with data from the oft-cited Alameda County Study and other investigations showing mortality rates higher for those who are socially isolated (Berkman 1995).

To consider the protective effect of social support in health care invites an interpersonal and relational perspective. Several investigations have examined the role of social support in marriage when a spouse is ill. Revenson (1994) synthesized results from a host of such studies. From this work, we learn that the quality of a marriage before the onset of illness predicts health outcome, with better marriages providing more support and experiencing the impact of the illness on the marriage as less negative. Also, especially with long-term conditions such as stroke and heart disease, spouses are often more stressed than are the patients themselves, having been challenged with their own emotional distress, sense of loss or sense of helplessness while meeting the patient's needs for practical assistance and emotional support. This dynamic appears to be more pronounced for wives than for husbands of the chronically ill, although more research on the role of gender in this context is needed (Revenson 1994, p.128).

Advancing this contextualized view of social support, Coyne (2000) discusses *relationship-focused coping*. From a long and impressive series of studies on the interactive nature of support, health and coping, he concludes that "appraisal [of stressors] is a social process, not a cognitive process" (Coyne 2000). In other words, factors such as faith, efficacy and expectation are all assessed through the filter of significant relationships in one's life. In studies with congestive heart failure patients, Coyne and his colleagues discovered that optimism on the part of the spouse predicted survival rates better than the patient's own optimism. Coyne identifies empathy as a relevant social skill in the health care context.

Early relationships may impact health in later life as well. In a 35-year-long prospective study of 116 men, Schwartz and Russek found that those who in college reported receiving more parental love and caring when they were children were in better health 35 years later, compared to the subjects who reported little parental caring. Eighty-seven per cent of those who rated their parents low on aspects of loving and caring suffered from illnesses such as coronary artery disease, hypertension and duodenal ulcers, while this was true for only 25 per cent of those who rated their parents high in parental caring. This remarkable effect was maintained even when the researchers controlled for other important factors such as family history of disease, smoking, marital status and age (Schwartz and Russek 2001).

Berkman (1995) recommends that interventions designed to supply social support when it is lacking aim to increase participants' sense of belongingness and the sense of competence. Note also that patients with chronic illness and their families have different needs than those with acute or imminently life-threatening conditions (Belar and Geisser 1995). There are several exemplary therapy programs to follow when offering support group work to medically ill patients, spouses, family members and caregivers. Among them, the celebrated work of David Spiegel and colleagues (Spiegel *et al.* 1989; Spiegel, Bloom and Yalom 1981) stands out, as they not only demonstrated psychosocial benefits of support group therapy for breast cancer patients, but also documented increases in life expectancy.

Mood and emotion

Mood, or emotional state, also impacts health. This occurs through direct physiological pathways (to be discussed in Chapter 3) and as a mediator of other factors such as coping and social support (Salovey *et al.* 2000). This is a potent area for dance/movement therapists to consider, because the modality has shown success with mood improvement in various populations (Brooks and Stark 1989; Cruz and Sabers 1998; Grodner *et al.* 1982; Kuettel 1982). Cohen (1997), writing from a DMT perspective, stated that emotions "serve to sensitize individuals to certain elements of a situation, and guide responses. Because emotions represent the integration of physiology, cognition, and memory, they must be viewed as pivotal in the stress–illness cycle" (p.2). In mind/body medicine literature, the emotions have generally been identified as negative (for example, anger, hostility, tension and fear) or positive (happiness, hope, optimism), although it is acknowledged that, in everyday life, feelings are mixed and experienced in paradoxical ways (Lazarus 2000). It is well established that sustained negative emotional states have negative health consequences (Sobel 1995). The research on stress, reviewed above, has tracked the many ways this transpires. More recently, researchers have turned their attention to the role of positive emotions and how they can be health enhancing (Folkman and Moskowitz 2000; Taylor *et al.* 2000).

In addition to the emotions named above, subjective well-being, creativity and optimal experience or "flow" (Csikszentmihialyi 1990) are all considered under the domain of positive psychology (Lazarus 2000). When related to health and illness, the concepts are linked to effective coping, supportive relationships, self-efficacy, meaning and motivation. Positive emotional experiences are not simply the obverse of negative affect. They can also occur even during the most difficult of times (Folkman and Moskowitz 2000). A key activity is *positive reappraisal*, or the "reframing [of] a situation to see it in a positive light" (Folkman and Moskowitz 2000, p.650), and it is part of making meaning out of traumatic or stressful events.

From a series of studies by Pennebaker and colleagues (Berry and Pennebaker 1993), we know that the expression of emotions, as opposed to the constraint of that expression, has health benefits. This is true for the expression of the negative emotions as well. Inhibiting the expression of negative emotions may in fact result in poor health outcomes (Salovey *et al.* 2000). Pennebaker's initial studies examined the health benefits of expressive writing for college students, using a number of behavioral as well as immunological indicators of health. They found that the disclosure of traumatic experiences through writing and the process of writing about one's feelings led to better immune system functioning (Pennebaker, Kiecolt-Glaser and Glaser 1988). Regarding nonverbal expression, they noted:

> a marked similarity between the relation of physiological response to the verbal disclosure of emotionally traumatic events, and to the disclosure of emotion via nonverbal expression. To the extent that the active ongoing

inhibition of nonverbal expression influences autonomic [nervous system] activity and places continual stress on the body, it would follow that nonverbal expressivity would also be related to health. Although less research is available regarding nonverbal expression, it is also likely that the nonverbal expression of emotion bears some relation to health status. (Berry and Pennebaker 1993, p.15)

Through analysis of the written material from study participants, they concluded that the organizing nature of the discursive written form was an important factor in yielding the health benefits. This form seems to have helped the students moderate the intensity of the emotions experienced and of the recruiting thinking functions, such as insight and the consideration of cause (Pennebaker 2000). According to Pennebaker, the enhancement of health through writing or speaking (in a clinical setting) about one's traumatic experiences comes from the combination of emotional and cognitive activities. The researchers recommended that the nonverbal therapies (naming dance, art and music therapies) would be enhanced by the inclusion of verbal expression in treatment sessions, and put out a call for more research on this question (Berry and Pennebaker 1993, p.18).

Krantz, a dance/movement therapist and psychologist, responded to that call with a valuable study that replicated the design used in several of the Pennebaker experiments, investigating the health benefits of expressive dancing, or "psychophysical expression" (1994). Krantz assigned 64 college students to one of three conditions:

1. dancing alone at home to express troubling feelings, thoughts or experiences

2. dancing as in the first condition, but then writing about the feelings expressed while dancing, and

3. a control condition wherein subjects participated in a non-expressive exercise task.

Krantz found that participants in the dance/write condition made fewer illness visits to the health center compared to those in the dance only condition and the exercise condition. Four months later, follow-up data showed a trend toward improvement in grade point average among participants in the dance/write condition, and this was not the case with those in the dance only and exercise conditions. Krantz noted that, in the short term, the subjects in both dance conditions reported an increase in physical symptoms such as headache and fatigue. With time, however:

the dance/write condition led to a decreased pattern of [physical] symptoms and dance alone led to decreased negative affect. Subjects in both dance conditions had positive evaluations of the study, even though they found it difficult to do movement. The psychological benefits of self-expressive action and dancing out troubling emotions included increased self-understanding and positive long-lasting effects of value and meaning from the experience. (Krantz 1994, p.i)

Dance alone did not bring about the positive health benefits in Krantz's study. She observed that the subjects in the dance conditions, generally unschooled in the art and craft of movement or dance expression, "experienced cathartic psychophysical release through dance, but they did not sufficiently articulate, organize and assimilate trauma to the extent they did in writing" (p.i). Krantz concluded that "a process of insight linked to emotional expression may underlie physiological changes that led to health benefits of confronting trauma" (p.i) and recommended the combination of dance and writing for health promotion.

When considering these findings for application in DMT, it is important to keep in mind the information about coping presented above. Recall that the simple venting of emotions is not an adaptive way of coping, and that staying with negative emotions for too long may initiate health-threatening processes associated with depression and depressed mood (Irwin et al. 1990). Dance/movement therapy focuses the attention on the body, heightening awareness of sensations. For medically ill people, this awareness is necessarily associated with heightened attention to symptoms. Note that the emotion of sadness also will increase the focus on oneself (Salovey et al. 2000). Reversing that feedback cycle, it is conceivable that patients in DMT, experiencing their bodies more acutely, could link feelings of sadness with the bodily sensations.

This occurred in my own practice when a woman with remitted lung cancer found herself crying during a simple guided relaxation exercise that focused on sensation. Her emotions could have been elicited through a process like this. She could not locate the cause of her sadness – she just felt sad and was unable to explain it. Initial experiences in DMT could temporarily increase any existing feelings of sadness and thus be uncomfortable for patients. Recalling Folkman and Moskowitz's (2000) discussion of positive appraisal, it would be important to help the patient openly discuss the sensations and to appraise them realistically. As advised by Pennebaker and by Krantz, catharsis is not enough and emotions need to be "worked through" using the organizing properties of spoken or written language.

Certainly, movement expression is not exclusively linked to emotion, and verbal processes are by no means purely cognitive in nature. The contrasts given in the work on emotional expression here may be linked to the fact that DMT research subjects are usually less experienced and facile with movement expression as a craft or language. Combined with the emphasis on sensation, the novelty may bring novice movers quickly to emotional experience. Conversely, in the verbal modality, with more skills and familiarity, people may move more easily into cognitive processes.

Spirituality and religion

Throughout this discussion, issues related to hope, belief systems, healing and meaning have arisen in a number of different contexts. Questions of spirituality and faith follow naturally from these phenomena. In cultures where healing and curing are conducted as religious rituals, the connection is obvious (Achterberg 1985; Rossi 1993) and dance is often involved (Halperin 1995; Hanna 1988, 1995; Katz 1984). For the same historical reasons that Engel (1977) alluded to, spirituality has long been cordoned off in conventional mental health and biomedical systems. However, in the last 20 years, researchers have brought the question back to the surface with information about the relationship of religion and spirituality to health, illness and mortality.

The distinction between religion, faith and spirituality is relevant here. Spirituality can be defined as "one's inward sense of something greater than the individual self or the meaning one perceives that transcends the immediate circumstances. 'Religion' may be described as the outward, concrete expression of such feelings" (Achterberg et al. 1994, p.8). Lukoff discussed the role of spirituality in mental health, using the phrase "spiritual emergencies", which are "crises during which the process of growth and change becomes chaotic and overwhelming" (Horrigan 2000, p.82). Certainly this describes the situation of an individual or family facing a newly diagnosed, chronic, or life-threatening illness or injury.

Nothing is proven unequivocally, but many studies suggest religious involvement may buffer impact of stress on physical and mental health, possibly through related psychosocial factors such as social support (Matthews et al. 1998; McCollough et al. 2000). The effect is not trivial. In their extensive meta-analytic review of 42 studies on the topic, McCollough et al. (2000) concluded that survival rates could be as high as 44 per cent higher for those who publicly practice their religion in a community, and that religion may be more of a health protective factor for women than for men. To ascertain the complex relationship between spirituality, religion and depression, Nelson and colleagues (2002) studied a group of terminally ill patients with cancer and AIDS using the FACIT Spiritual Well-Being Scale. In their sample of 162 subjects, they found a negative correlation between spirituality and depression, yet a positive correlation between religiosity and depression.

Lukoff cautioned practitioners who use mind/body interventions to know fully the spiritual or religious origins of the methods, because mind/body work will evoke issues of spirituality or transcendence (Horrigan 2000). I observed this myself in a small DMT support group for parents of hospitalized children, conducted in the open lounge area of a hospital family resource center. Asked to develop a movement phrase to represent something that she herself needed, one mother assumed "prayer position hands" (fingers lengthened and palms together), closed her eyes and began rocking. Clear that she needed prayers, she moved quickly into a religious and prayerful state. It was important that I acknowledged her action as both a spiritual communication and a movement expression.

Cohen (1997) addressed both meditation and DMT as mind/body interventions, which by using breath and sensation, bring about a sense of wholeness and connection and link to healing and spirituality. She offered provocative and important questions about the juxtaposed relationship of stillness (as practiced in meditation and many conventional religious contexts in the U.S.) and movement (as guided in DMT): "Does the harmony of mind–body processes occur in both movement and stillness?... What are the differences and similarities between stillness and movement in altering levels of awareness and integration?" (p.3). As Cohen concluded, these are questions for future research, and when answered will apply directly to DMT work at the bedside with patients who have very little movement capacity.

Imagery

There is plentiful evidence that imagery influences health. In relation to the issue of stress, Baum (1990) reports on research findings that "chronic stress is related to the frequency or intensity of images and thoughts about past stressors" (p.669) and that "psychophysiological aspects of an event may be duplicated in imagined representations of the event" (p.671). Rossman (2000) states that "imagery is the interface between what we call body and what we call mind" (p.16). To do justice to the vast body of knowledge on imagery and health is beyond the scope of this volume, but several concepts and studies are highlighted because they can inform the practice of medical DMT. Body image is a central construct for DMT and this will be examined. Patients' imagery about their bodies and their disease will also be considered. Finally, the use of imagery techniques will be reviewed. Because health-relevant imagery often occurs during altered states of consciousness, including creative and movement states like those generated in DMT sessions, the dynamics and induction of such states will also be discussed.

Body image and body imagery in illness

Dance/movement therapists address body image in their work, both for assessment and in treatment interventions (Franklin 1979; Serlin *et al.* 2000; Wise and Kierr Wise 1985). It is a complex psychophysical phenomenon (Schilder 1950) and there is no single accepted definition of the construct (Dosamantes 1992). However, it is commonly understood that the body image is the mental representation of the body that includes sensations, memories, values and attitudes about the body. It is a dynamic rather than static process. Vamos (1993) considered body image "central to the discipline of psychosomatic medicine" (p.164) and outlined four dimensions of body experience affected by chronic physical illness: comfort, competence, appearance and predictability. In more acute illnesses or injury, the body image is disrupted, with psychic attention redistributed to the affected body zones (Goodill and Morningstar 1993). There is often a temporary or permanent partial loss in body functioning. Sometimes body parts or organs are lost or changed and the body self-image must adjust. In addition, those who are close to that individual must adjust too, and the ill or injured person needs to cope with the reactions of others to his or her body. Enormous contributions of mental and emotional energy are required for the individual to adjust to the changes or loss (Cash and Pruzinsky 1990). Fisher and Cleveland (1968) are among the major researchers of this process, notable for their neurological study of the well-known "phantom limb" syndrome, wherein a patient who has lost a body part to surgery or injury continues to receive sensations as though the limb or other part was still present.

Patients with various ailments and diseases report vivid and poignant body imagery that is connected to the illness and the body's experience with it. For example, gout, a painful and acute form of arthritis, is described by its victims as "like matches", "setting the joint on fire", "the devil gnawing at my big toe", and "like walking on my eyeballs" (compiled and cited in Tatum-Fairfax 2002). Yardley (1996) related the experience of a woman with multiple sclerosis whose body image changes extend to the dimensions of space and time: "the bathroom which was 'near' becomes 'far', while the workplace may become unattainably distant; stairs and spaces become the barriers instead of the means to translocation; the pace of living may be slowed while, paradoxically, the future dwindles and disappears" (Toombs 1992, as cited in Yardley 1996, p.498). The body image in illness is easily and frequently represented in drawings or other artwork

(Malchiodi 1999a, 1999b). Given these characteristics of body image, it is arguable that DMT, with its focus on psychophysical and emotional integration, is a preferred modality for helping a patient make the adjustments to a changed or impaired body in illness or after injury (Berrol, Ooi and Katz 1997; Dibbel-Hope 2000; Serlin *et al.* 2000). Wise and Kierr Wise (1985) give a simple and apt explanation: "Body image problems can be successfully treated with movement therapy because it is in action and interaction that the inner, feeling self and the outer, physical self can get to know one another and work together to fill mutual needs" (p.176).

In groundbreaking research with cancer patients, Achterberg and Lawlis (1978) investigated the prognostic value of imagery. In studies on their Image–CA assessment, patients with metastatic disease are first guided into a relaxed state, then asked to visualize three aspects of their internal experience: the cancer/tumor and its cells, the immune system and the (current or previously received) cancer treatment. The patient then makes a drawing with all three components of the imagery. Following this, the patient is interviewed about the imagery and other thoughts regarding the illness and the treatment. Material from both are scored on several dimensions: the vividness, strength and activity of cancer cells and the white blood cells (WBCs); the vividness and effectiveness of the treatment; the size of the WBCs; the size and number of cancer cells; the choice of symbolism; the integration of the whole imagery process and the regularity of imagined positive outcome. At two months follow-up, the Image–CA assessment scores were the most significant predictor of disease status: more so than WBC counts, hormonal factors, and other psychological factors of denial, locus of control or the level of self-investment (Achterberg 1985, pp.186–7). With 93 per cent certainty, the imagery predicted the patients whose disease went into remission during those two months, and with 100 per cent certainty the imagery predicted death or marked deterioration in health status (p.189). It was the *interaction* of the three imagery components – disease, immune system and treatment – that accounted for most of the effect, although some symbols seem to have prognostic implications. Specifically, images of cancer that included ants or crustaceans, or very destructive elements such as fire or poisons, were associated with poor prognosis, as were mechanical treatment images like axes, picks or vacuum cleaners. Images of the immune system that were associated with good prognosis included big animals in action such as bears or dogs, and powerful warriors like Vikings, or "white knights" (Achterberg and Lawlis 1978, pp.95– 6).

Given the potential for imagery to influence both psychological states and the progress of disease, a host of therapists and researchers from a variety of disciplines have developed clinical interventions that employ imagery. Imagery is considered an essential ingredient in many mind/body medicine approaches and falls into the healing aspect of the healing/curing distinction outlined in Chapter 1. It is important for patients who use imagery for healing to understand that they did not cause their own illness through negative imagery or pessimistic thoughts. The unfounded sense of guilt that may accompany such a belief could itself compromise efforts towards adaptive coping (Harpham 1994).

Dance/movement therapists routinely employ imagery in their work with mental health and medically involved patients, usually allowing imagery to arise from the group's or individual's psychophysical expression (Mendelsohn 1999; Serlin 1993, 1996b). There are differences in the way that DMT usually integrates imagery and how it is used in some other mind/body practices. In some other mind/body methods such as hypnosis (Belsky and Khanna 1994; Yapko 1990) the therapist will often provide the image, using knowledge from human anatomy and physiology along with findings like Achterberg's, to create the visualization sequences. Some believe that imagery for healing should be very specific, and others advocate for general healing imagery (Rossman 2000). In DMT, the ongoing movement process elicits kinesthetic and mental images in the patient, which are at some point vocalized, verbalized, or represented in the form of the movement. Then together the patient(s) and therapist improvise, interact and shape the image towards the salient interpersonal or intrapersonal meaning (Sandel 1993a).

Also, in a number of other mind/body practices, such as hypnosis or GIM™ (Guided Imagery through Music) (Summer 1990), the patient will remain in relative stillness with an internal focus in a relaxed state. In this regard it is interesting to consider findings that "imagery flows best when the motor system is not actively competing for the brain's attention" (Bakan 1980, as cited in Achterberg 1985, p.188). In a pilot study to explore a similar question Finisdore (1997) found that participants in Authentic Movement™ sessions experienced more imagery and performed less movement when first inducted into a relaxed hypnotic state. Dance/movement therapists who integrate other forms of mind/body medicine approaches may find themselves switching between their familiar active and interactive imagemaking processes, as described by Sandel, to formats where the patient is experiencing body imagery in more passive and receptive states. The merits of each in a medical DMT context have yet to be compared empirically.

State change

When imagery is employed in any of the ways described above, the individual's state of consciousness is altered from everyday awareness. This may entail a relaxed state in which the health-beneficial relaxation response (Benson 1975) is elicited, a trance state in which the awareness is deliberately redirected away from external realities (Rossi 1993; Temes 1999) or mobile states as in dance healing rituals (Halperin 1995; Hanna 1988). All change the individual's perceptions of the self and the immediate surroundings and are believed to open neurological channels in a way that permits psychophysical change. Active, conscious engagement of breath is common in the induction of altered states for healing purposes. In general, short, fast, shallow breathing is linked to anxious states and the fight–flight response. Mind/body healing methods, including the more active ones like DMT, often cue the patient to deepen and expand the breathing pattern. Montello (1996), writing from a music therapy perspective where breath is also important, acknowledged the breath poetically:

> The breath is the life force which flows in and through the body–mind allowing us to move, grow, and fulfill our soul's purpose. The breath is the link between the body and the mind. Inhaling, we are taking in life; exhaling, we are expressing life. When we are breathing deeply and our inhalations and exhalations are evenly timed with no pause in between, we are in a state of perfect balance and harmony. As our breathing becomes more rhythmic, the mind automatically follows suit. And with that steady rhythm comes a feeling of security and power that allows us the ability to move forward with confidence and one-pointed vision. (p.44)

The theory of State Dependent Learning Memory and Behavior (SDLMB) (Rossi 1993) helps explain the mechanisms of mind/body medicine's use of altered states. Simply put, the theory posits that learning achieved in a certain state is best recalled when again in that state. It is for this reason that students are advised to study for exams in physical situations that resemble the test-taking environment.

The process operates to threaten and to enhance health. For example, memories of traumatic experiences are easily triggered by trace elements of the circumstances in which the trauma first occurred, and the memory may trigger the same fight–flight response and behavioral patterns that were experienced with the original trauma (Baum 1990). The experience is encoded, and state-bound. Conversely, when people are in a relaxed state of openness to change and make insights or realizations that are valuable to their well-being (e.g., towards more self-efficacy, congruence, or peacefulness), they are predisposed to recreate those conditions within themselves in the future. Rossi wrote:

> according to this view, what we usually experience as our ordinary everyday state of awareness or consciousness is actually habitual patterns of state-dependent memories, associations and behaviors. I have conceptualized

"creative moments" in dreams, artistic and scientific creativity, and everyday life as breaks in these habitual patterns. (Rossi 1993, p.53)

Hypnosis and some forms of meditation induce this type of "change-friendly" altered state. Meditation can be broadly defined as "an intentional regulation of attention from moment to moment...[in which] a passive attitude is maintained" (Kutz et al. 1985, p.2). Chang (1997) has blended mindfulness meditation, as a body-based approach, with DMT, to derive an integration called "mindful moving" – where "taking embodiment into action relates the [sic] sensitized internal process to the environment" (p.152). Hypnosis is variously defined and often misunderstood. Here are a few definitions by leaders in the method, provided by Temes (1999):

> Dr. Milton Erickson (1901–1980), one of the pioneers of hypnotherapy and the founder and first president of the American Society of Clinical Hypnosis, defined hypnosis as a natural, everyday experience of unconscious learning via successful communication.

> ...Dr. Herbert Spiegel defines hypnosis as the condition that occurs when the patient feels as if he is floating, feels as if he is simultaneously "here" and "there" (i.e. achieves dissociation), and is able to maintain focused concentration while being open to suggestions... In 1993, the Division of Psychological Hypnosis of the APA defined hypnosis as a procedure wherein changes in sensations, perceptions, thoughts, feelings or behavior are suggested. (p.3)

A clinical hypnosis session usually proceeds with an induction first and then the hypnotic suggestions (Temes 1999), a sequence that is roughly analogous to the warm-up into theme development sequence of a standard DMT session (Chaiklin and Schmais 1993).

Ernest Rossi (1993), who collaborated for many years with Milton Erickson, has applied clinical hypnosis to mind/body healing and developed an integrated psychobiological framework for it. He observed that good hypnosis subjects tend to be good placebo responders and to have strong right hemisphere dominant characteristics such as creative traits (pp.34–5). Recall that body image has been localized to right brain functioning, and a pattern emerges to suggest the type of patient who might benefit most from mind/body techniques that employ altered states and the use of imagery. Interestingly, in a study of the absorption factor, a trait connected to hypnotic responsiveness, Goodman and Holroyd (1993) found that DMT trainees score higher in absorption than do students in other fields. Absorption is a "state of receptivity or openness to experiencing in the sense of readiness to undergo whatever experiential events, sensory or imaginal, that may occur with a tendency to dwell on, rather than go beyond, the experiences themselves and the objects they represent" (Tellegen 1981, as cited in Goodman 1993, p.43). This may reflect a natural proclivity for absorption among those who seek to enter the field, and it may also be an effect of training for DMT. It follows logically that people who are, either constitutionally or by training, inclined to "absorb" the felt experiences of others would seek a profession where these traits are valued. Whether similar tendencies characterize the more responsive consumers of DMT has not been researched, but given the shared attributes between DMT and hypnosis (altered state, use of breath, use of imagery, creative processes and intention towards change), it is a question worth pursuing.

Rossi's particular version of mind/body healing through hypnosis is a "content free" form of trance experience in which the therapist does not introduce metaphors, but lets them arise within the patient so that what he calls "preconscious implicate processing" can occur (Rossi 1999). The method also involves "ideo-motor" movement, a small and usually gestural movement on the part of the patient because, according to Rossi (1999), it is the behavior *with* the thought that makes the method effective. The movement is invited during the "suggestion" portion of a session, and is a way to active problem solving (while in trance) and internal conflict resolution in the patient.

The use of medical hypnosis spans the entire diagnostic spectrum. Belsky and Khanna (1994) reported on a small but successful study of a self-hypnosis intervention for children aged 7–18 with cystic fibrosis. Pre-to-post-test changes in the treatment group were significant for locus of control, health locus of control and self-concept. Between group differences in changes from pre-to-post-test were significant for increases in peak expiratory flow rate, a measure of respiratory functioning. Successful treatment with medical hypnosis has been reported with asthma (Wagaman 1999), cancer pain and side effects of chemotherapy (Levitan 1999).

Rossman (2000) described imagery work with a wide range of adult patients, many of whom suffer from ailments easily exacerbated by stress and sometimes considered somaticization problems (Wickramasekera 1998). These problems are readily responsive to imagery (Rossman 2000, p.17). Rossman's patients learn self-guided imagery practices that they use independently as well as in session, which seems to be prescription for enhanced self-efficacy.

The discussion of imagery leads us to theories about mental and physical states that lead to emotional, psychological and behavioral change. Therapists of many persuasions seek to create these states within their patients. These "states for change" are variously known as liminal states, "flow", play states, trance states, transformational states and creative states. Kubie (1958) conceptualized the "preconscious state" as attended by flexibility of image, free play, invention, simultaneous perception of many things, overlapping meanings. The preconscious state is fluid and mentally swift, opening the individual to new discoveries and to the perception of similarities. Kopp (1972/1988), an eclectic psychologist, drew on Carl Jung's thinking when he wrote that the psychotherapist's job is to "provide a dreamlike atmosphere" (p.5). Anthropologist Victor Turner (1967) sees in liminal states, induced with trance and ritual during rites of passage and other times of change, the conditions for profound change and healing in the individual. Csikzentmihalyi (1990) described the state of flow as an optimal experience in which, "people are so involved in an activity that nothing else seems to matter" (p.4) and "when consciousness is harmoniously ordered..." (p.6). This is akin to playful, spontaneous, improvisational states, sensitively described by Nachmanovich (1990) who perceived the value of a "play space" where without fear of criticism one can experiment with unconscious material, as in psychotherapy "in which we enjoy perfect confidentiality that enables us to explore the deepest and most troubling matters in our lives" (p.69). Nachmanovich singled out the creative activities of the arts as a process that "resembles the best in psychotherapy" (p.185). This is consistent with Winnicott's (1971/1985) concepts of the transitional space in therapy, which recreates the original "playground" between the child and the primary caregiver. This playground, the space between, is where therapeutic change occurs. "To get to the idea of play," Winnicott instructed, "it is helpful to think of the preoccupation that characterizes the playing of a young child. The content does not matter. What matters is the near-withdrawal state..." (p.60). He continued:

> The general principle seems to me to be valid that psychotherapy is done in the overlap of the two play areas, that of the patient and that of the therapist. If the therapist cannot play, then he is not suitable for the work. If the patient cannot play, then something needs to be done to enable the patient to become able to play, after which psychotherapy may begin. The reason why playing is essential is that it is in playing that the patient is being creative [and]...it is only in being creative that the individual discovers the self. (p.62)

The ever-changing, ongoing nature of dance movement manifests all of these features in therapy. For the literal and apparent reason that it is impossible to be moving and still at the same time, movement states are essentially liminal. Shapiro (1999) explores the movement phrase, a small unit of behavior, as an organized microcosm of behavior and personal style (see also Davis 1991; Dell 1970). She proposes that the movement phrase is itself a liminal phenomenon and recommends interventions at the level of the phrase, attending to dynamic qualities, nuances and sequences. Laban (1980) observed "transformational drives" in human movement: constellations of movement qualities, or Efforts, that evoke an intensity of experience. They are labeled *vision drive, passion drive* and *spell drive*, the last of which is "hypnotic" (Bartenieff 1980) and seems to "radiate a quality of fascination" (Laban 1980, p.81). Halperin's research (1995) identified movers in trance during healing rituals manifesting the transformational drives, suggesting that there is an observable change in movement state when the mental/spiritual/ physical state is also altered. These movement states have been studied for their mythical and fantasy properties (Bartenieff 1980) and considered part of the process of change as well (Zacharias 1984). States that could be theoretically related to trance are those described by Laban as the *spell drive*, the *vision drive*, and the *dream inner attitude*. This emphasis on the quality, rather than the quantity, of movement is another feature of DMT that allows for easy adaptation of clinical methods to situations where mobility is reduced.

Hanna (1988) examined the altered states produced in dance healing rituals from the physiological angle. She noted that an altered state typically induced prior to dance rituals through methods such as sleep or food deprivation, and in this state the dancers enter the typically prolonged, high energy, multi-sensory experience of the ritual. Thus, homeostasis is deliberately disrupted and when exhaustion sets in, a cascade of metabolic reactions occur, leading to a changed perception of the body and the surroundings, and a transformational or liminal state (see Turner 1967).

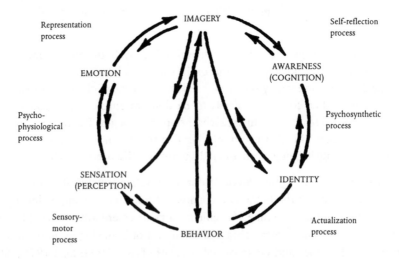

Figure 2.1 Rossi's modalities of mind/body communication and healing. From Rossi, E. L. (1993) The Psychobiology of Mind/Body Healing, revised edition, New York and London: W. W. Norton and Co. Copyright ©1993 Ernest Lawrence Rossi. Reproduced by permission of the publishers.

Rossi (1993) provides an integrated schema for the dynamics of thought, feeling, sensation and action in mind/body healing and psychological change (see Figure 2.1). An individual can enter the cycle at any point, and transition to any of the other states or processes via the pathways Rossi has hypothesized. In addition, he noted that each modality has state-dependent features and has its own "genius", manifested in a form of psychotherapy, in relation to these modalities of experience (1999). DMT seems to have its genius in the area of sensorimotor processes at the sensation/perception node of the cycle. Note that in Figure 2.1 this leads easily to emotion, imagery and behavior, all of which are key ingredients in DMT healing processes (Schmais 1985).

This chapter has traversed the domains of health psychology and mind/body research to lay a theoretical foundation for the practice of DMT with medically ill people and their families. The reader is equipped with basic knowledge of the prevailing constructs and concerns in behavioral medicine and emerging concepts regarding treatment. Under each of the processes discussed in this chapter are physiological events that involve all of the body's systems. To lay the foundation for an integrated mind/body framework for medical DMT, the next chapter introduces scientific information and theory.

CHAPTER 3

The Science behind Medical Dance/Movement Therapy

Well, can we add a cubit to our height
Or heal ourselves by taking conscious thought?
The spirit sits as a bird singing
High in a grove of hollow trees whose red sap rises
saturated with advice...

Close your eyes, knowing
That healing is a work of darkness,
That darkness is a gown of healing...

From "Ode to Healing," by John Updike[1]

This chapter presents research from the scientific disciplines of psychoneuro-immunology, neuroendocrinology and studies from various medical science areas. There is an emphasis on research with implications for understanding the mind/body integration as it is viewed and employed in the practice of dance/movement therapy (DMT). Explanatory research for the mechanisms of DMT, whether in conventional mental health applications or in relation to total health, will likely come from interdisciplinary efforts with the fields of neuroscience, physiology, psychoneuroimmunology (PNI) and movement science (an academic branch of physical therapy). PNI is an interdisciplinary field concerned with relationships among the nervous, endocrine (or hormonal) and immune systems with regards

---

1   From *Facing Nature* by John Updike, copyright © 1985 by John Updike. Reproduced by permission of Alfred A. Knopf, a division of Random House, Inc., and Penguin Group UK.

to stress, emotions, personality, cognition and other psychological variables (Jemmott 1985). The science is "devoted to studying the two-way relationship between the nervous system and the immune system" (Friedman, H. Klein and Friedman 1996, p. i). Work in these areas has proceeded rapidly in the past two decades. Most of what is known was discovered first in animal model studies and then extended to work with human subjects. Little if any of it has been concerned directly with DMT processes or outcomes. Nonetheless, aspects of this body of research support DMT's premises regarding the reciprocal nature of the mind/body connection and the inherently curative properties of creative movement expression (Schmais 1974, 1985). Taken as a whole, these findings provide a rationale for utilizing DMT in a general health care context.

The interaction of the central nervous system and other body systems is nearly simultaneous (Pert *et al.* 1985), making it impossible to impart the true nature of the dynamic in time-bound writing. Systems interact in bidirectional and multiple ways; there are redundancies in the systems that maintain homeostasis; and feedback networks that signal and regulate immunologic or hormonal responses create paradoxical situations within the body. To harness these complexities, the discussion will begin with the brain, with the now familiar stress phenomenon that includes the hypothalamic–pituitary–adrenal pathway, and a brief review of hormonal involvement. From there, we will follow the pathway to the immuno-logical system, which enables the consideration of direct effects of psychological and emotional status on health and disease. A look at selected research on the con-nections between the musculoskeletal system and the brain will bring the discus-sion towards implications for DMT, which functions chiefly through that system. The chapter concludes with a review of treatments and a speculative discussion on the possible mechanisms by which expressive and creative movement processes might influence physical health. As with the concepts presented in Chapter 2, the coverage of these many and complex processes is necessarily brief and elementary. In-depth discussions are beyond the scope and intent of this volume, but are refer-enced throughout the chapter for the reader who wants more detail.

The stress response

The human nervous system is composed of two main anatomical branches: the *central nervous system* (CNS), consisting of the brain and the spinal cord, and the *peripheral nervous system*, consisting of the nerve fibers that interact with the body's tissues and communicate with the CNS. The CNS system has two functional branches: the *somatic nervous system*, consisting of the motor neurons that supply the skeletal muscles, and the *autonomic nervous system* (ANS), consisting of the nerve fibers that innervate smooth muscle, cardiac muscle and glands (Sherwood 1997, p.112). The ANS is further divided into the *sympathetic nervous system* (SNS) and the *parasympathetic nervous system* (PNS). It is here in the ANS where the stress response and its sequelae occur. While the somatic nervous system is generally under voluntary control, the ANS usually operates involuntarily. There is emerging evidence of voluntary control of some ANS functions, to be discussed below in relation to mind/body interventions.

The concepts of homeostasis and self-regulation are key to understanding the ANS (see Chapter 1), and Harvard physiologist W. B. Cannon (1932) explained *homeostasis* as a process of the human body interacting with the environment:

> This personal individual climate, which we carry with us, must not greatly change if we are to continue to be effective. For constancy of the internal environment, therefore, every change in the outer world, and every consider-able move in relation to the outer world must be attended by a rectifying process in the inner world of the organism... The chief agency of this recti-fying process is the sympathetic nervous system. (p.267)

The body perceives a stressor (i.e., danger, shock, fear, trauma, or grief) as a threat to homeostasis, and the CNS makes a quick response, known as the *fight–flight response*, trying to return to what Cannon called its steady state. Environmental stimuli become chemical signals in the form of hormones and complex molecular structures that travel through the body, connecting and configuring with each other and target organs. Nerve fibers involved in the stress response emanate from the thoracic and lumbar regions of the spine (see Figure 3.1). The reactions observed in the fight–flight pattern are the result of action on target organs as the system readies the person for intense physical action. As the body works to mobilize energy and increase the blood supply to skeletal muscles there is an increased consumption of glucose, increased blood pressure and increased heart rate. The digestive system, immune system and urinary activity decrease so as not to siphon the body's resources from the task at hand: survival. As the peripheral muscle warms with the increased blood supply, increased sweating occurs. Pupils dilate and there is an overall sense of arousal. All of this can occur within a matter of seconds.

The PNS works with the SNS to regulate responses to stress. Herbert Benson first described the action of the PNS as the "relaxation response" (Benson 1975; Friedman, R. *et al.* 1996). "The relaxation response is the behavioral and physio-logical opposite of the fight-or-flight response" (Friedman, R. *et al.* 1996, p.365). Nerve fibers from the cranial and sacral regions of the spine are involved in para-sympathetic response. Manifestations of this complement to the fight–flight response include the slowing of breath rate and heart rate, and increasing digestive activity. The PNS brings the body back from aroused states such as the *stress response*.

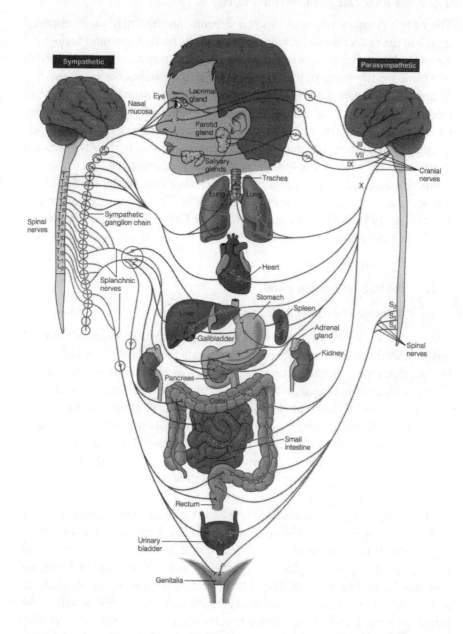

Figure 3.1 Innervation of organs by the SNS and PNS. From Sherwood, L. (1997) Human Physiology, From Cells to Systems, *3rd edition, by Sherwood. © 1997. Belmont, CA: Wadsworth Publishing. Reproduced with permission of Brooks/Cole, a division of Thomson Learning.*

The HPA axis and its hormonal activity

The body's complex response to stress depends on the finely tuned chemical signals of the endocrine, or hormonal, system of the body. A common analogy for the endocrine system is that it interacts with the nervous system the way the pedals on a piano modify the quality of the notes played; some hormones are *excitatory* in nature and stimulate activity, others are *inhibitory* in nature and regulate or modulate other reactions. Hormones are not traditionally classified as neurotransmitters, but they are acting similarly to neurotransmitters, or chemical messengers, in the processes related herein. The initial pathway in the ANS response to stress is SNS's use of the *hypothalamic–pituitary–adrenal* (HPA) axis. This is a neuroendocrine pathway wherein brain structures stimulate the production of hormones and the hormones act on target organs. This chain of events, which Hans Selye (1956/1976) later elaborated as the General Adaptation Syndrome, develops in three stages:

1. the alarm reaction

2. the stage of resistance and

3. the stage of exhaustion (Selye 1956/1976, p.1).

The syndrome begins with the *hypothalamus*, a subcortical structure made of specific nuclei and associated fibers that lie beneath the thalamus. The hypothalamus regulates many homeostatic functions, such as temperature control, thirst, urine output and food intake. It forms a link between the nervous and endocrine systems of the body and through its many connections with the limbic system in the midbrain; it is also extensively involved with emotion and basic behavioral responses (Sherwood 1997). The hypothalamus receives information from the external environment through sensory receptors that "perform the function of *transduction,* [meaning] that they convert one form of energy to another" (Winters and Anderson 1985, p.71).

In the fight–flight response (see Figure 3.2) the neurons in the hypothalamus secrete *corticotropin-releasing hormone* (CRH). CRH travels through the bloodstream a very short distance to the anterior pituitary gland, a two-lobed structure, where it stimulates the pituitary gland to synthesize and release another hormone: *adrenocorticotropic hormone* (ACTH). ACTH is carried through the bloodstream downward to the *adrenal glands,* which sit atop the kidneys, where it stimulates the cortex (or outer layer) of the adrenal to release a glucocorticoid called *cortisol.* Cortisol is a protein, commonly known as the *stress hormone* (Sherwood 1997). The hormones in the HPA cascade are all *peptides,* made from amino acids. There are other hormones released by the hypothalamus to the anterior and posterior

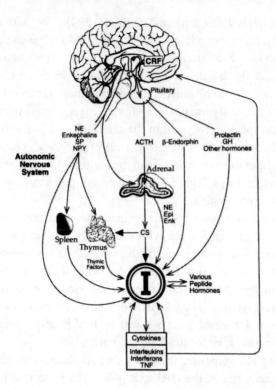

Figure 3.2 The ANS response to stress. From Dunn, A. J. (1996) "Psychoneuroimmunology, stress and infection" in H. Friedman, T. W. Klein and A. L. Friedman (eds) Psychoneuroimmunology, Stress and Infection, *Boca Raton, FL: CRC Press, p. 31. Reproduced with permission.*

pituitary glands, and other hormones released from them; however, this discussion is limited to the stress response and its health effects and thus the CRH–ACTH–cortisol system. Cortisol travels in the blood to the target organs, which then change their activity to respond to the stress, as described above. This is the stress pathway that uses the pituitary gland. Normally, increased cortisol will appear in the bloodstream approximately 30 minutes from the onset of a stressor (Herbert and Cohen 1993).

There is another sequence, known as the *sympathoadrenomedullary system* (sometimes referred to as the SA system or the SNS pathway) that involves a direct activation of the *adrenal medulla* (the core layer of the adrenal gland) by nerves emanating from the spinal cord. The stimulation causes the adrenal medulla to release the excitatory hormones *epinephrine* and *norepinephrine*, also known as the *catecholamines*, into the bloodstream (Dunn 1996) in a reaction that is faster than the HPA axis pathway (Herbert and Cohen 1993). The adrenocortical and adrenomedullary hormones all act on target cells and on the immune system.

As noted above, there are also numerous neural connections between the hypothalamus and the limbic system of the brain, which processes emotions. Thus, the HPA cascade can be initiated by internal stimuli from other parts of the brain as well as external stimuli. In addition, stress causes increased synaptic release of norepinephrine (NE) within the cerebrum and "NE cell bodies in the brain stem send collaterals to widespread areas of the brain" (Dunn 1996, p.29). Thus the CNS responds to stress locally in the brain, and peripherally throughout the body in parallel ways. Figure 3.2 shows both pathways and indicates the impact on the immune system.

As in all homeostatic functions, the sympathetic and parasympathetic systems act constantly and in complement with each other, enabling us to respond to stressors as needed and shutting off the response when it is no longer necessary. Hormones such as cortisol that are associated with health threats or decreased immune function are not intrinsically negative substances; on the contrary, as will be seen in the next section, they stimulate the immune system at everyday levels. Catecholamines and cortisol pose a threat to health only when too much is released and circulating, or for too long a duration.

In the relaxation response, there is a hypothalamus-initiated generalized decrease in the activities of the HPA axis (Rossi 1993), so that in the ongoing dynamic balancing of SNS and PNS systems, the PNS is ascendant. Interestingly, the HPA axis also stimulates the production of pain-blunting chemicals, the *endorphins* and *enkaphalins*, substances that are known to create sensations of pleasure and to enhance immune system functioning (Achterberg 1985). The discussion of DMT for chronic pain in Chapter 4 will address the role of these endogenous opioids further.

The *limbic system*, a midbrain collection of structures, processes emotions and has a role in memory. LeDoux (1993) identified the *amygdala*, a limbic system organ, as responding to fear and encoding memories connected to fearful events. Summarizing a series of animal model studies on emotional learning, he asserted:

> ...the neural mechanisms of emotion and memory have long been thought to reside side by side, if not in overlapping structures, of the limbic system. However, the limbic system concept is no longer acceptable as an account of the neural basis of memory or emotion and is being replaced with specific circuit accounts of specific emotional and memory processes. Emotional memory, a special category of memory, involving the implicit (probably unconscious) learning and storage of information about the emotional significance of events, is modeled in rodent experiments using aversive classical

conditioning techniques. The neural system underlying emotional memory critically involves the amygdala and structures with which it is connected. (LeDoux 1993, p.69)

The amygdala also integrates motor functioning: "Within the amygdala, the lateral nucleus (AL) is the sensory interface and the central nucleus [is] the linkage with motor systems involved in the control of species-typical emotional behaviors and autonomic responses" (LeDoux 1993, p.69). Consider this with Winters and Anderson's reminder that "neural activity in the CNS is in a constant state of flux and the organism's reaction to a stimulus is, in part, determined by its state at the time the stimulus arrives (1985, p.79). One can take from these a suggestion that people who are undergoing or about to undergo stressful or frightening experiences such as invasive medical procedures or getting a diagnosis would be well advised to enter those situations in a steady state, with a CNS that is calm and unencumbered by heightened SNS activity. Inasmuch as these experiences are by nature frightening, supportive interventions to reduce anxiety and fear may be indicated as advisable.

Pathway to the immune system

The immune system is key to the maintenance of homeostasis. "Disregulation, and hence poor physical and/or emotional health, occurs when there is attenuation, distortion, disconnection, or dissattention to feedback from the external environment or the internal milieu" (Winters and Anderson 1985, p.67). Most of the time the immune system works with the nervous and endocrine systems in finely tuned attention to the internal mileau, adjusting to ANS changes and interactions with the external environment. As in any true system, numerous interdependent relationships between components and overlapping feedback loops enable the immune system to perceive and disable foreign (non-self) matter that would infect and harm the body: virus, bacteria, allergens, fungi and transplanted tissue as well as altered, abnormal cells of the self (i.e., cancer cells). Immunity is a highly complex process that is now understood at the sub-molecular level, and a full presentation of the system is well beyond the scope of this book. For the present needs, a cursory overview will be augmented by information that elucidates the mechanisms of mind/body interventions. This discussion is drawn from works by Sherwood (1997), Parham (2000) and Cotman et al. (1987). Many of the terms used in immunology are borrowed from language we use to describe human behavior, reflecting the dynamism and intelligence of the system. These rich descriptors are an anthropomorphizing of the elements and reactions however, and it is important to keep in mind that the communication in the system is entirely through chemicals, movement of cells around the body, and changing structures in molecules and cells. Much of this is accomplished with binding sites and receptors on cells, making for key-in-lock fits between elements. For extensive and accessible coverage of the immune system, see Parham (2000).

The immune system operates in three ways:

- with physical barriers that prevent the entry of pathogens to body tissues

- with the mechanisms of the innate, or natural, immunity which makes an initial and non-specific attack on infections

- with the highly specific responses of adaptive immunity that usually result in long-term memory of specific infectious agents.

Physical barriers include the skin and the mucosal surfaces of the body in contact with the environment. The *mucosal surfaces* are lined with *cilia* to block entry to the body's tissues and enzymes to break down and disable the pathogen itself. When the barrier defense system is breached, the innate and adaptive aspects are mobilized.

The immune system is composed of:

- *lymphoid tissues* that are distributed around the body: importantly in the bone marrow, the small intestine, lymph nodes and the thymus gland

- blood components: *white blood cells* (WBCs) or *leukocytes*, and the many substances that exude from and interact with the WBCs.

Several types of WBCs form in a progression of developments beginning as the hemopeoetic stem cells of the bone marrow. *Monocytes* or *macrophages* eliminate infectious organisms by engulfing and then decomposing them. Another type of WBC, the large *natural killer* (NK) cells destroy altered, potentially cancerous cells that are found even in healthy bodies. *Neutrophils* are WBCs that circulate in the blood and travel to sites of invading pathogens. *Basophils* and *eosinophils* are also types of WBCs, smaller in number. T-cells mature in the *thymus* (the T stands for thymus), and perform one of two functions. *Cytotoxic T-cells*, also called *CD8+ cells*, actively kill cells that have been invaded by foreign antigens. They release toxic chemicals that perforate the cell's walls and then send in enzymes to destroy the cell. *Helper T-cells*, also referred to as *CD4+ cells*, make and secrete proteins called cytokines. Helper T-cells are the primary target of the *human immunodeficiency virus* (HIV). *Cytokines* and *chemokines*, sometimes called *lymphokines*, are chemical messengers which induce, inhibit or otherwise regulate the actions of the WBCs. They are named according to their function. An *interleukin* is a factor produced by one leukocyte to act on another – IL-1, IL-2, IL-6 and IL-12 all figure in the neuroimmune pathways studied in mind/body interactions. For example, IL-2 is a growth factor for T-cells. *Tumor necrosis factors* (TNF) assist in inflammatory processes, and the *interferons* (INF) assist with resistance to viral infections. *B-cells,* so named because they are derived from the bone marrow (Janeway and Travers 1996), are WBCs that function primarily to form and secrete *immunoglobulins,* or antibodies. Immunoglobulins (the Igs) are part of the initial, innate response to infection. These may sit on the surface of a B-cell where they recognize and bind to antigens, or they may circulate in the bloodstream as *antibodies.* Antibodies will adhere to an antigen with a high degree of specificity, which means that antibodies can modify their structure to fit and thereafter remember a given antigen. Immunoglobulin-A, secreted in both blood and saliva, is an oft-used indicator of immune system responsiveness in PNI studies.

Ader (1996) observed that "all immunoregulatory processes take place within a neuroendocrine milieu that is demonstrably sensitive to the influence of the individual's perception of and response to events occurring in the external world" (p.15). Figure 3.2 shows that the release of hormones such as those involved in the stress response stimulates the immune system, also demonstrating the feedback loop from immune system components to the central nervous system. Fehder and Douglas (2001) summed up the interactions between the immune and nervous systems in three categories, the second two of which make vital use of the endocrine system.

> In particular, these relationships take the form of immunologically derived cells that are resident in the central nervous system (CNS) that under special circumstances take part in immune reactions in the CNS. Furthermore, the direct innervation of immune system associated organs such as the spleen and lymph nodes and the response of immune cell traffic in these organs to nerve signals such as neuropeptides show the close connection between the immune and nervous system. Finally, neurons and immune cells secrete and bear receptors for many of the same chemical messengers that include cytokines, neuropeptides and hormones. This evidence supports the existence of a common chemical language between these body systems. (Fehder and Douglas 2001, p.229)

This is the bidirectional aspect of the mind/body connection at a biological level. Ader provided details, explaining how "activation of the immune system is accompanied by changes in hypothalamic, autonomic, and endocrine processes, and by changes in behavior. For example, cytokines influence activation of the HPA axis – and, in turn, are influenced by glucocorticoid secretion" (Ader 1996, p.15). Lower levels of glucocorticoid secretion are essential for stimulating a normal immune response but in high doses (as in acutely stressful events) have inhibitory effects on the immune system (Dunn 1996). The catacholamines also seem to inhibit NK cell activity (Dunn 1996, p.33). Some endocrine substances stimulate the immune system, including the pituitary-derived hormones *prolactin* and *melatonin* (which is the hormone that brings on sleepiness). Another interesting feedback loop is demonstrated in the fact that infections themselves bring about internal and behavioral changes that mimic responses to psychologic stressors. Specifically, "infections activate the HPA axis and the SA system, and increase the synaptic release of NE and 5-HT [the neurotransmitter serotonin] in the brain" (Dunn 1996, p.35).

Effects of psychological and emotional status on health and illness

Observable interactions between the components of the neural, endocrine and immune systems are important because they point to the body's fluctuating ability to remain healthy. Researchers caution that these are only indicators, and it is the actual presence of disease, distress and/or health that is most relevant (Irwin *et al.* 1990; Kaplan 1990). Further, most studies have clarified associations between components, but not necessarily causation.

> In many instances, it is impossible to determine whether the immune-modifying variable exerts its primary impact indirectly via the stress response or directly on the immunologic parameter being studied. Both direct and indirect influences are probably being exerted. It is also important to note from the outset that many of the studies reveal correlations, and that cause and effect relationships can only be implied. (Hall *et al.* 1994, p.184).

Different models have been hypothesized to chart the influence of feelings, thoughts and behavior on health. Herbert and Cohen (1993) hold that "negative events (stressors) lead to negative affective states (distress) that then relate to alterations in human immunity" (p.364). Elaborating on this, others have delineated a pathway beginning with a stressor to distress to an underlying mechanism to immunity to health (Keller *et al.* 1994). For PNI research, the stress/distress is the psychological or psychosocial aspect, the neuroendocrine activity manifests the underlying mechanism, and from the immune system changes, health or disease results (Keller *et al.* 1994, p.218).

Each link in the chain proposed above has been established, but to date there is no definitive study or series of studies that proves the entire model. Thus, it is best to stay aware that "neither a genetic predisposition, exposure to a pathogen nor the experience of a stressful event is able, by itself, to trigger a predictable progression of disease. Instead, each of these contributes to the psychological and physiological responses of the organism. These combined responses ultimately determine the balance point between good health and disease" (Hall *et al.* 1994, p.201). In this section, notable studies linking emotion to immunity and health are reviewed.

In the 1990s research by neuroscientist Candace Pert and colleagues gained the attention of the lay public and contributed to mainstream appreciation of the mind/body connection. Pert and colleagues (1985) found that a special class of proteins, *neuropeptides*, can *chemotax* (or travel) between the emotion-mediating limbic system of the brain, receptors in the spinal cord, the gastrointestinal system and the WBCs of the immune system. These chemical messengers are synthesized in both the CNS and by immune system cells, and there are receptors for the neuropeptides in all of these other "nodal points" (Pert *et al.* 1985, p.821s). Thus, the physiological substrate of emotion is a phenomenon of the brain and the body, with simultaneous actions throughout. This revises even the biopsychosocial concept of interacting systems to the notion of a single system or "psychosomatic network" (p.820s). Pert's work is basic science, much of it conducted using animal models. Nonetheless, she has been able to draw out the implications of this molecular level work in terms of human feelings and lifestyle (Pert 1997), and the work is applauded by scientists, the media and patients alike (Moyers 1993).

Irwin and colleagues (1990) compared 36 matched pairs of hospitalized depressed patients and nondepressed control subjects to examine the ways that depression and severe stressors both impact the neruoendocrine and immune systems. They found that immune changes during depression imitate some medical symptoms and vice versa. Specifically, "both major depressive disorder and the presence of threatening life events in control subjects are independently associated with a 50% reduction of natural killer (NK) cytotoxicity" (p.28). The association was maintained even when controlling for age, alcohol and tobacco use, which are known moderators of immune functioning (Irwin 1999). Recall that stress stimulates the immune system, but in chronic or extremely threatening stress, the minor stimulatory benefit is offset by these troubles. Chronic stress predominates the subjective experience of depression and creates several negative consequences for the immune system. *Glucocorticoids*, the stress hormones, decrease the production of IL-2 and other cytokines, leading to sluggish or inadequate stimulation of the system. Production of the cytokine INF (interferon) also decreases, and this interferes with the activity of the NK cells, thereby reducing resistance to viral infections. The production of antibodies by B-cells is inhibited by stress, with antibodies against herpes viruses and hepatitis B most clearly affected (Glaser and Kiecolt-Glaser 1998).

The demands of caregiving for Alzheimer's disease or AIDS patients, the death of a spouse and divorce or separation can also lead to a decreases in immune system functioning, with individuals' responses mediated by the many psychological factors discussed in Chapter 2 (Schneiderman and Baum 1991).

The neurotransmitter *serotonin* also has a role in the relationship between depression and health. *Cerebral serotonin* is reduced in depression, and it is also reduced by stress. Low levels of serotonin are associated with increased aggression and with the subjective experience of distress. Conversely, increased *functional serotonin* is associated with increased calmness and feelings of serenity. Dunn (1996) noted that the changes are more commonly observed following protracted stress. *Melatonin*, the sleep-related hormone released as part of the circadium rhythm, is also thought to be an immunity enhancer. Sleep is disturbed in most physical illnesses, and also in depression. Coupled with the other immune depleting aspects of depression, the disruption of sleep and subsequent decrease in melatonin release introduces additional health risks (Irwin 1999). In depression, there are also behavioral changes that may invite poor health. This may occur through the poor self-care, nutrition and exercise habits attendant to depression, or, as Herbert and Cohen observed, "behavioral adaptations may themselves lead to physiologic changes that lead to additional immune alteration" (Herbert and Cohen 1993, p.374).

The common cold is a condition encountered by almost everyone. A head cold is hardly life threatening, but because of its relatively short duration and benign health consequences, it is easily researched for PNI purposes. Bovbjerg and Stone (1996) reviewed a series of studies on the common cold and relate good evidence for a causal relationship between either increases in undesirable events or decreases in desirable events within a three- to five-day period preceding onset of cold symptoms. Many of the studies track the secretion, concentration and functional activity of the antibody *Secretory IgA* during that time frame. Salivary S-IgA is thought to reduce the risk of infection by interfering with viral attachment to epithelial surfaces. IgA is used as a marker of immune system activity and to collect it from salivary glands is a non-invasive and relatively inexpensive procedure (Jemmott and McClelland 1989). Other studies exploring treatment effects of mind/body interventions have observed increases in S-IgA and linked it to beneficial effects.

With evidence for the negative effects of stress and depression on health well researched, questions about the possible positive effects of pleasant states have recently surfaced (Billings *et al.* 2000). There is currently insufficient scientific evidence to provide a complete model such as that for stress and the HPA and SA mechanisms, but some studies have made promising discoveries. Futterman and colleagues (1992) conducted a fascinating study examining the impact of brief emotional states on the immune system. Professional method actors were asked to induce in themselves a variety of moods: anxiety, depression, happiness and a neutral control state. The actors' "performances" in the affect states were video-taped and then an impartial rater correctly identified the intended state. The activity of cytotoxic T-cells, helper T-cells and NK cells were analyzed from blood samples drawn between affect state inductions. All three of the affect states produced more immune system variability than did the neutral state, but they found more variability during the high arousal states (anxiety and happiness) than in the depressed and neutral states. The positive/negative valences in emotional tone did not seem to effect the immune system differently. From this, the researchers concluded:

> ...it is possible that arousal, not the specific "positive" or "negative" affect condition, caused the immunological variability observed. Future studies with experimentally induced affect should consider the role of emotional arousal and intensity. (Futterman *et al.* 1992, pp.236–7)

With the possibility that negative and positive emotions both influence health indicators, the field is open to examining the impact of positive emotional states on health. This more expansive research agenda bodes well for a field like DMT where patients experience a full range of emotions, and sometimes have fun.

Breath: Physiology, emotions and movement

Respiratory disorders, ranging from the common cold to asthma to cystic fibrosis, have been the concern of mind/body specialists and researchers. Perhaps this is because the breath is a cardinal indicator of life itself, or because the act of breathing puts the external environment in immediate contact with the internal body environment. The physiology of respiration suggests a possible mechanism for this. The simplified discussion that follows is taken from Sherwood's text (1997) and equips the reader to use breathing techniques and imagery that is physiologically accurate.

The *medullary control center* located in the brain stem sets up the alternation between inhalation and exhalation, modulates the rate and depth of breathing, and governs other breath functions such as speaking or sneezing. An inhalation begins when the *phrenic nerve*, originating in the cervical region of the spine, stim-ulates the *diaphragm* to contract and descend in the *thoracic cavity*. This activity simply increases the cavity's volume in the vertical dimension and air flows in as the lungs expand to fill the available space. Supplementally, the external *intercostal muscles* between the ribs contract and expand the thoracic cavity in the side–side and sagittal dimensions. Exhalation is a passive process during quiet breathing – it is accomplished by the relaxation of the diaphragm and subsequent shortening of the thoracic cavity space. In forceful exhaling, the internal intercostal muscles contract to narrow the space of the cavity, and *abdominal muscles* contract to push the diaphragm upwards as well. The *oxygen* (O_2) delivered by inflowing air travels through a series of branching and ever smaller airways until, at the thin walled *alveoli*, it diffuses into the bloodstream through the comparably thin walls of the *pulmonary capillaries*. There, the waste product *carbon dioxide* (CO_2) diffuses in the opposite direction, from the blood to the lung cavity. Once in the bloodstream the O_2 is carried to tissues where it is transformed into energy. In *musculoskeletal muscle*, this transformation occurs in a process called *oxidative phosphorylation*. The energy producing process relies on both oxygen and glucose products, namely *glycogen*, a glucose polymer. The production and expenditure of energy in the muscle tissue figure into the mechanisms for dance in health, as described by Hanna (1988) below.

Asthma is a common reactive airway disease characterized by acute constriction of the bronchial tubes in the lung. "It is presumed that a genetic basis predisposes an individual to bronchoconstriction" (Mrazek and Klinnert 1991, p.1014), but some asthma attacks can be precipitated by emotions or distress, and sometimes predictably. Mrazek and Klinnert reviewed findings that "negative emotions related to interpersonal interactions have the greatest potential for triggering wheezing in stress-sensitive asthmatics" (p.1023).

Paradoxically, *bronchoconstriction* could be triggered by the relaxation response of the ANS. In addition to the other patterns described above, the SNS activates *bronchodilation*, opening airways to bring in more oxygen when needed for physical exertion and quick action. Conversely, in the usual reciprocal dynamic of the SNS and PNS, stimulation of the nerves to the respiratory apparatus by the PNS brings about *bronchoconstriction* (Sherwood 1997, p.208–209). The *vagus nerve* is the major cranial nerve of the PNS and innervates muscles in the organs of the thoracic region including the lungs (Sherwood 1997, pp.141–2). "Bronchoconstriction in asthmatics might result from an imbalance in sympathetic and parasympathetic regulation. This has been referred to as parasympathetic dominance" (Mrazek and Klinnert 1991, p.1024). For the mind/body specialist who will employ relaxation techniques with asthma patients, it is important to keep the potential for this physiological reaction in mind.

Brain waves, muscle activation and states of consciousness

The previous chapter identified the altering of consciousness as an ingredient in mind/body healing processes. The physiological correlates to states of consciousness are part of the mind/body integration, and research findings on these links may shed light on the mechanisms of DMT. *Consciousness* can be defined as:

> subjective awareness of the external world and self, including awareness of the private inner world of one's own mind – that is, awareness of thoughts, perceptions, dreams, and so on. The following states of consciousness are listed in decreasing order of level of arousal, based on the extent of interaction between peripheral stimuli and the brain: maximum alertness, wakefulness, sleep (several different types), coma. (Sherwood 1997, p.143)

These levels can be measured in humans with EEG, or *electroencephalography*, using terminals on the scalp that pick up cerebral cortex activity. EMG, *electromyography*, measures muscle tone using surface terminals placed either on the skin directly above the muscle of interest (Basmajian and Blumenstein 1980), or on a needle inserted into the muscle fiber.

Connections between EMG and EEG have been discovered in sleep studies and with subjects in awake states as well. Three brain wave rhythms are of interest when considering the potential relationships between imagery, movement and health status. The descriptions will use the terms *synchronous* and *dissynchronous* to characterize brain wave activity. Note that synchrony means that the activity at the neuronal synapses is in a resting state or in low activity. Desynchronized EEG waves indicate a high level of synaptic activity. Usually, we have synchronized rhythms when asleep and desynchronized waves when awake (Winters and Anderson 1985).

Alpha waves occur during awake, relaxed and innattentive states and have attributes of low frequency and rhythmic or synchronous activity. *Theta waves* are just a little slower than in the alpha pattern, are also present in relaxed states and predominate in trance and hypnogogic states (Freeman and Lawlis 2001). *Beta waves* occur during awake, attentive and mentally active states. They have the attributes of low amplitude, high frequency and dissynchrony (or *arrhythmia*) (Winters and Anderson 1985). They also occur during REM, also known as *paradoxical sleep*, when dreaming occurs. It is hard to arouse the sleeper from beta-wave sleep, but sometimes the sleeper awakes spontaneously from this state (Sherwood 1997, p.144). In this state, there is a profoundly decreased muscle tone on EMG and no movement. *Delta waves* occur during slow-wave sleep, the first stage of a sleep cycle when dreaming is rare and it is easy to arouse the sleeper (see Sherwood

1977, p.144). Delta waves are of high amplitude, low frequency and sychronous, rhythmic attributes. In slow-wave sleep, there are delta waves and decreased muscle tone (as measured by EMG).

There are implications for health associated with all three types of brain activity. Irwin *et al.* (1990) found that sleep disturbance was coincident in their depressed and highly stressed subjects, noting that loss of "slow-wave sleep has been found to alter the secretory response of IL-1, important in the stimulation of NK cells" (Irwin *et al.* 1990, p.28). Achterberg's research on the imagery of cancer patients included an investigation of neurological correlates to imagery states. They found that during visual imagery, alpha waves were suppressed, especially for inexperienced imagers, and that for these subjects, alpha-wave suppression was a better predictor of imagery experience than was self-report by the subjects. Moreover, when there was an increase in the use of symbolism in the imagery, there was a decrease in alpha waves recorded on EEG, especially with symbolism about cancer cells being attacked (Achterberg and Lawlis 1978, pp.144–6).

The current technology available to researchers does not permit accurate EEG measurement of people who are in full body movement. However, with voluntary, gestural position-holding actions, an association between EMG readings and the magnitude of beta-wave activity, as measured by EEG, has been established (Halliday *et al.* 1998). Researchers have also found that EEG patterns are similar when a subject imagines a small hand movement as when the subject actually prepares to execute that movement (Pfurtscheller and Neuper 1997). Specifically, similar patterns of "event related desynchronization" (Pfurtscheller and Neuper 1997, p.65) of both alpha and beta waves occur during motor imagery as during the preparatory phase of movement (p.66). A potential implication of these findings is that some EEG (cortical) activity might be inferred from EMG readings during awake states. This lends new import to early studies in which measurement of Laban-described movement features was achieved using EMG technology (Bernstein and Cafarelli 1972; Chatfield 1998; Hunt 1973).

Because Laban Movement Analysis (LMA) concepts will appear through this volume, a brief introduction to Laban's theory is warranted. This review of Effort theory is drawn primarily from the works of North (1972), Dell (1970) and Bartenieff (1980). Laban and colleagues observed the dynamic quality of human movement and described this as an "inner impulse to move" (Bartenieff 1980). Laban used the German word *antrieb* for this, which translated best to the English term *effort* (Laban 1980). The Efforts are ubiquitous and naturally occurring qualities that are seen in both functional (instrumental) action and in expressive movement; in both intentional, conscious usage and in an out-of-awareness, spontaneous way. They are seen in postural or gestural activity and occur when we are alone or interacting with others. The Efforts are categorized into four main factors, known as motion factors: *flow, space, weight* and *time.*

Each motion factor has two elements, presented as polarities, but on a continuum, with gradations of intensity and neutrality. Laban categorized the Efforts into two main clusters, according to the *polarities,* or Effort *elements* named above. According to Laban, the indulging elements are the qualities that yield to time, space, weight or flow. They are *free flow, lightness, indirect space* and *sustainment.* In opposition to this, the qualities of *bound flow, strength, direct space* and *quickness* have a resisting quality, and are known as the *fighting elements.* In everyday movement of normally functioning adults, it is rare to see a single Effort. In most adult human activity, Efforts occur in combination. Combinations of two Efforts are known as *inner attitudes,* or *inner states,* and reflect the internalized mental state of the mover. Combinations of three Efforts are known as *drives.* The three *transformational drives* were mentioned in Chapter 2. The fourth, the *action drive,* combines an element of *space,* an element of *time* and an element of *weight.* These combinations are often used in task activity. They are devoid of the *flow* component (which is associated with emotion), tend to convey a clear impression of the mover's skill, and the movement tends to be suitably adapted to the demands of the task at hand. When moving in *action drive* one is engaging the attentional/thinking, intentional/sensing and intuitive/deciding functions in oneself.

The Bernstein and Cafarelli study (1972) provided an electromyographical validation of Laban's Effort theory showing that distinct EMG tracings are produced during each of the eight action drive Effort combinations. Bernstein and Cafarelli used the limb movement of a single subject and a panel of expert observers to verify the presence of the movement combinations under study. Hunt (1973) observed that emotional content manifested in changed EMG patterns only when her subject thought about communicating the emotion, and not when simply thinking about an emotion-laden event. The changes were different for negative and positive emotional imagery. Inferring from her findings, Hunt recommended to dance/movement therapists the encouragement of movement states that correlate with pleasant affects.

While not oriented to the Laban system, Streepay and Gross (1998) used kinematic research techniques to quantify differences in neutral, fear and anger expressions in dancers, and measuring range of motion and velocity as parameters of interest. Range of motion in the lower spine and shoulder areas during both of the emotional-expression patterns for fear and anger differed significantly from the neutral state but were not markedly distinguishable from each other. Velocity differed between emotions, with the lowest velocities in neutral movement and the highest velocities in anger. The Streepay and Gross study demonstrates that:

- differences between emotional and neutral expressive intentions can be measured quantitatively, and

- these differences manifest in movement.

Two other pilot studies contribute pieces to the puzzle of the movement/ brain/health dynamic. Sakamoto (2001) compared four conditions: a resting baseline, imagery, movement and movement/imagery combination using three dependent variable: heart rate, EMG of the corrugator muscle (roughly located on the forehead between the eyebrows), and self-report for mood, in a sample of 15 depressed university students. Imagery was intended to bring about a pleasant state, and the movement instructions were for gentle, releasing movements. EMG activity was elevated, though not significantly, in the combination condition when compared to the other three. Heart rate (an indicator of SNS activity) was significantly reduced in all three experimental conditions, with the lowest heart rate in the imagery/movement combination condition. Self-reported anger followed a similar pattern, with significant reductions in imagery and movement conditions, and a greater reduction in the imagery/movement combination. Curiously, *hedonic tone* (a positive emotional parameter) was highest in the baseline resting condition, possibly due to some discomfort with the novel imagery and movement tasks. Sakamoto did not observe the dynamic qualities of the subjects' movement, so inferences regarding Effort elements are not possible from this study.

An exploration of the relationship between mental imagery and the production of Efforts in movement was conducted by Dayanim (1998). Forty normal school-aged children were told "image stories" with instructions to act out the stories in movement. Dayanim found that, with 75 per cent reliability, commonly used imagery language for Laban's eight basic Efforts was successful in eliciting the intended movement quality.

Clearly, imagery is an active mental process. In several mind/body healing practices, it is often introduced into consciousness following the induction of a relaxed state (Halprin 2000; Rossi 1993; Rossman 2000). However, it is fair to assume that the movement states induced in most DMT methods would likely be accompanied by beta waves and, since imagery is used, would probably involve alpha-wave suppression in inexperienced imagers. Thus, using brain waves as a criterion, movement is not necessarily relaxing to the CNS when it is happening (people may achieve a relaxed state afterwards, but not during movement). Other indicators – heart rate and self-assessment of anger – indicate beneficial aspects of movement combined with imagery (Sakamoto 2001). The question arises: what is happening neurophysiologically in interventions where people transition from relaxed alpha-wave type states, as in relaxation, to the alpha-suppressive use of imagery (when moving or not) and the beta-wave alertness of movement in inter-action? And what might be the health implications, if any, of those changes? Certainly, CNS arousal occurs with most DMT and mind/body interventions. Recall from Chapter 2 that Rossi's methods of hypnosis for mind/body healing actively employ imagery, and some physical movement as well. He explains how the alternating cycles of relaxation and CNS arousal encode the positive cognitive and emotional discoveries made in such altered states (Rossi 1993). Perhaps the same kind of process is operating in DMT as well. Taken together, the research presented in this section suggests a rationale for investigating a link between imagery, movement, cortical activity, ANS reactions and health indicators.

Interactions with the musculoskeletal system

Returning to information about the breathing process, we now see that upon arousal by internal or external emotional or perceptual cues, the fight–flight response quickens and increases the delivery of oxygen and glucose products ingredients for energy – to the voluntary muscles. Without release, when physical reactions to the stress response are thwarted or otherwise disallowed, the glycogen and glucocorticoids need to be reabsorbed into the system. When the system is overwhelmed by intense or unremitting stressors, normal homeostatic processes may be insufficient for returning the organism (the person) to healthy baselines. This may set the stage for some of the cardiovascular and other health problems associated with the constraint of expression and chronic tension (Sherwood 1997, p.672). Hanna (1988) observes correctly that dancing and other physical activities "use up" these chemicals, clearing the system and giving the PNS opportunity to modulate neuroendocrine responses. Hanna also noted "vigorous dancing induces the release of endorphins thought to produce analgesia and euphoria" (p.12). Unlike simple exercise, dance/movement activity adds the benefit of emotional expression, ostensibly tied to the emotion or perceived threat that triggered the fight–flight response to begin with. The tension that compels emotional expression is dissipated, leaving the patient in the relational context of the therapy, aware of feelings and perceptions, but having discharged the bio-chemical products of the stress response.

This is where Rossi's (1993) concept of state-dependent learning, memory and behavior informs medical DMT. DMT processes may bring to the surface difficult memories or conflicts in one's life, but the modality, with its physical and relational features, enhances the body's own homeostatic potentials. Patients in DMT do experience the state-bound challenges of their lives in a very real and felt sense. Re-learning occurs when the previously threatening states associated with thoughts, memories and feelings are brought into the therapeutic milieu where patients actually practice their own mind/body's abilities to manage arousal and stress. This line of thinking recalls Johnson's (1987) and Burgess's (Hartman and Burgess 1988) discussions of trauma processing. When addressing psychosocial aspects of medical conditions, the trauma is usually related to diagnosis, medical treatments, body image and functional adjustments, family adaptations, and issues concerning death and dying.

Berrol (1992) identified several other neurophysiological aspects of DMT that have implications for health. *Rhythm*, she explained, is "an attribute of central nervous system patterning" (p.25) and influences ANS responses to organize and regulate the intensities of physiological, emotional and behavioral events. Berrol called for research that will explore "whether the coupling of rhythm with selected movement intensities impact on bioaminergic systems or arousal mechanisms" (p.24). Findings from inquiry like this may enable the identification of mechanisms of DMT as it relates to the physical health/illness spectrum. It is posited that the intersection of motion and emotion is localized at the *basal ganglia* or *basal nuclei,* which are situated in the cerebral cortex. In 1974, Bartenieff presciently proposed that the Efforts are crystallized by the basal ganglia. Future research will need to pursue an integrated understanding of the potential interaction between emotion, the limbic system, ANS events, the basal nuclei and Effort production in movement expression.

Mind/body interventions

Mind/body interventions attempt to harness the natural reciprocity between thought, emotions, physiology and immunity to influence health in a positive way, by either reducing detrimental factors or introducing and enhancing beneficial factors. These factors are derived from research on the many modifying variables discussed in this and the previous chapter. Most successful PNI interventions reported in the literature employ some form of relaxation with or without guided imagery, with combinations of hypnosis and relaxation common as well (Kiecolt-Glaser and Glaser 1992). Other components may include music, cognitive methods to help patients modify their expectations or attitudes towards the disease or the treatment, or social support (i.e., group treatment formats).

As Berrol (1992) noted, music accompanies many DMT sessions and so some of the health benefits conveyed through music may be accessible to patients in

DMT. Music listening has been shown to reduce blood cortisol levels in depressed teenage girls (Field *et al.* 1998) and to enhance salivary S-IgA production during dental procedures for female patients (Goff, Rebollo Pratt and Madrigal 1997). Participation in group music therapy, including music listening and improvisational techniques, can increase salivary IgA levels and decrease salivary cortisol levels in hospitalized adult cancer patients (Burns *et al.* 2001). In an elaborate multidisciplinary investigation, group drumming in music therapy was shown to enhance several indicators of immune functioning: increased NK cell activity, enhanced lymphokine (cytokine) stimulated killer cells, and an increased ratio of DHEA (an antiglucocorticoid agent) to cortisol in the blood (Bittman *et al.* 2001).

Imagery techniques have been researched with a variety of medical populations. Cohen (1991) found that guided imagery could reduce hypersensitivity to ragweed pollen and symptom reduction in allergic subjects. In laboratory studies, Jasnoski (1994) has suggested that there may be image specificity in immune reactivity, meaning, for example, that salivary IgA antibody and not other immune components will increase on suggestion with specific IgA imagery, and the converse will be true when, for example, the imagery is directed to helper T-cells in the blood.

Esterling (1991) found that interventions with relaxation and exercise improved immune resistance to both the Epstien-Barr virus and a herpes virus for men undergoing the stress of HIV status diagnosis. Fawzy and Fawzy related findings by Schneiderman, Antoni, LaPierriere and Fletcher (1990, in Fawzy and Fawzy 1994) that after a 10-week stress reduction program with relaxation, exercise, coping and self-efficacy foci, HIV-positive men showed significant improvements in mood and in helper T-cell levels. Burns (1996) compared the immune effects of relaxation training and humor groups among juvenile offenders. He found that both methods enhance the immune system's response, measured by salivary IgA concentrations, but that the humor groups produced the largest effect.

Darby's (1990) study discovered that self-hypnosis practiced over a three-week period could enhance helper T-cell counts, suppressor T-cell counts and NK cell counts in a normal university sample. In a well-designed study, Whitehouse *et al.* (1996) researched the benefits of self-hypnosis for medical school students undergoing the stressor of academic demands, including final exams. This kind of stress has been shown to suppress the immune system (Kiecolt-Glaser and Glaser 1992). The Whitehouse group measured reductions in anxiety and distress in the experimental group, but only the self-reported quality of the relaxation itself enhanced immune functioning (evidenced by increased number and activity of NK cells) (p.257). The one DMT study that has examined effectiveness with test anxiety (Erwin-Grabner *et al.* 1999) suggests that DMT may also help to reduce academic stress. To date, research on immune system effects of DMT, neither in relation to academic stress nor any other threat to physical health, have yet to be published.

Fawzy and Fawzy (1994) tested the efficacy of a controlled six-week psychoeducational and group support program for patients with malignant melanoma on psychosocial and immunological parameters. In short, group participants made significantly greater improvements on several mood measures, in coping strategies and immune functioning (three types of NK cells). Post-treatment differences in response between treatment and control groups were maintained at six-month follow-up. Gruber *et al.* (1988, in Hall *et al.* 1994), report on a year-long study with adult patients with metastatic cancer. Using a single-subject multiple baseline design, they tracked several psychological and immune measures while patients engaged in a program of relaxation and imagery. Participants showed steady and sustained increases in two antibodies (IgG and IgM), NK cell activity and in IL-2 levels. Subjects also reported an increased sense of control as the study progressed (attributing this to a midway presentation of encouraging study data to them), and evidenced a sense of optimism as well.

Critiquing these and similar findings, Hall and colleagues (1994) speculate that guided imagery itself may not be the causative agent for the positive changes observed, but rather that "engaging in the behaviors associated with guided imagery is conducive to good health" (p.193). Another review of psychosocial interventions (Hall and O'Grady 1991) concludes with a proposal that two main factors account for the health benefits of those treatment approaches: relaxation and expectation. Expectation is one's belief in the efficacy of a treatment (Hall and O'Grady 1991, p.1077) and its potency is connected to optimism, the strength of the clinical relationship, belief systems and mechanisms underlying the placebo effect. Relaxation has its own clear impact on the ANS and immune system, and treatments that include relaxation are tapping into these mechanisms. To this they added the concept of physiological toughness, which suggests that "exposure to intermittent stressors reduces basal levels of sympathetic nervous system arousal, but results in a strong level of sympathetic arousal in response to subsequent stressors" (Hall and O'Grady 1991, p.1077). The authors highlighted the compatible idea that "relaxation works by reducing SNS arousal if one considers that it is a sequence consisting of relaxation followed by arousal that is important (Dardik 1986)" (Hall and O'Grady 1991, p.1077). This echoes and supports Futterman's (Futterman *et al.* 1992) laboratory-based findings regarding emotional arousal and immune variability, as well as Rossi's (1993) clinical use of alternating relaxation and psychoemotional arousal in hypnosis for mind/body healing.

This chapter has briefly described major scientific principles and findings that can inform the practice of medical DMT. Basic to many of these is the role of the ANS as a regulator of the body's internal state. ANS activity is manifest in all body systems in direct and indirect ways. Research on how emotions and behaviors play a role in immune system functioning is ongoing. Studies of the musculoskeletal system and its relationship to both expressive movement or mental states and cerebral activity were also reviewed. Relationships between these systems and overall health have yet to be definitively linked with DMT processes; based on the existing science, speculations can be made regarding the possible mechanisms by which expressive and creative movement processes might influence physical health.

Possible mechanisms for DMT in physical health

Throughout this chapter, evidence has been presented that suggests several possible mechanisms for DMT's potential to enhance or maintain health and alleviate the discomforts or symptoms of disease or injury. These notions are theoretical and tentative, derived from seeking similarities between features of DMT and those of related and better-studied mind/body interventions in the literature reviewed.

DMT, being a form of moderate exercise, confers the same benefits. Hanna's work proposes a stress reduction model for DMT, as it acts to attenuate deleterious effects of the fight–flight response and its sequelae. The explanatory models involving behaviors and health habits might also speak to the DMT process, because in DMT, patients actively rehearse behavioral change and revise their experience of the state-bound emotions that interfere with full functioning. The development and exploration of imagery is central to the practice of DMT (Sandel 1993a) and inasmuch as imagery itself may produce physiological change, this may be operative in DMT as well. Neuroscience findings linking brain wave activity (represented by EEG readings) to muscle activity (measured by EMG) and mental imagery indicate how the imagery pathway might work. Caldwell (2001) has recently discussed the role of dopamine pathways in the link between emotion, movement and creative activity. That the pathway through the emotions is part of the puzzle is feasible because DMT has previously demonstrated effectiveness with improving mood and decreasing anxiety (Brooks and Stark 1989; Cruz and Sabers 1998; Ritter and Low 1996).

These and other research priorities will be considered further in Chapter 7. Bovbjerg and Stone advised "it is appropriate that early investigators focus on establishing [a] phenomenon before attempting to explain how it works" (1996, p.206). Fortunately, dance/movement therapists specializing in medical applications have done just that and through casework, pilot projects and a handful of empirical studies are exploring the ways DMT can improve quality of life and physical symptoms. The chapters to follow relate their endeavors and their stories.

Part II

Applications of Medical Dance/Movement Therapy

Prologue

I see, Kiwi,
You have wings
But cannot fly.
Yes, that is true
But...what do you do?
Everything else.

Old Japanese poem[1]

Early on, dance/movement therapy (DMT) positioned itself in the field of mental health with a primary focus on mental illness, developmental impairments and behavioral disorders. However, since the inception of the field, dance/movement therapists have made forays into the medical arena with case reports and pilot research studies dating back at least to the early 1980s (McKibben 1982, as cited in Seides 1986). In Part I, psychological and scientific foundations for medical DMT were presented. Part II reviews representative medical DMT work to date and embraces the wide variety of theoretical approaches, conditions addressed, and clinical methods reported in the field. In Chapter 4, non-oncology applications are covered. Because cancer-related work is well developed in the field, it will be covered separately, in Chapter 5. Chapter 6 discusses related applications of DMT with families and caregivers of medical patients, and with death, dying and bereavement work.

DMT sources for Part II include conference presentations, doctoral dissertations, Masters' theses, published and unpublished literature along with new

---

1   From *International Arts Medicine Newsletter* (1997), Vol.12, no.3. Reprinted with permission.

material from this author's own clinical work and interviews with several other medical DMT specialists. For this author, a motivating question has been "how, if at all, are conventional DMT techniques adapted to meet the needs of primarily medically ill people?" Therefore, in the pages to follow I have described clinical methods that are familiar to dance/movement therapists practicing with mental health populations, as well as methods that are uniquely suited to the medical context. Suggestions for clinical methods and training exercises can also be found in Chapter 9.

CHAPTER 4

Dance/Movement Therapy in General Medical Care

This far-ranging content will be organized around the following broad categories of recipient populations: adult patients, and child and adolescent patients. These divisions are somewhat reductionistic, and two caveats apply. First, pain is an over-riding aspect of many medical conditions and could easily be addressed from that more general perspective. However, there are some conditions in which pain is the central symptom and focus. For the sake of expediency, issues regarding pain and pain relief for adults will be discussed in the context of the pain syndromes. When dance/movement therapy (DMT) is used for pain relief in other medical conditions (such as cancer, or post-surgical recovery) the same principles as are involved with pain syndromes are relevant and can be adapted to those needs. Second, issues surrounding death and dying are addressed later, in Chapter 6. Obviously, those issues may be significant to medical patients at any stage of an acute or chronic illness. Still, facilitating or supporting the processes of dying and bereavement requires particular knowledge and skill of the therapist, and the discussion of them is thus given its own context.

Adult patients

Pain

Pain, like stress, is a whole body phenomenon. In part, pain uses the same stress system pathways that are implicated in the health problems described earlier in this volume. Writing from a constructionist point of view, Yardley (1996) defined the experience of pain and suffering as "an intersubjective phenomenon, constantly negotiated and redefined by sufferers and their immediate social contacts (family, doctors, employers) in the wider context of their cultural and socio-economic circumstances" (p.491). Kaplan (1990) reviewed evidence on the relationship between pain and stress, concluding with the suggestion that pain and suffering are *distinct*. The relationship between the two may be seen in a sequence wherein the initial pain perception leads immediately to pain evaluation, and this to an emotional reaction. Over time, the pain can take on meaning and this is where suffering begins. The emotions of suffering are hopelessness, help-lessness, depression and frustration (Barsky and Baszender 1998).

Pain itself has adverse health effects: long-term changes in the nervous system, depression of the immune system, decreased mobility, decreased lung functioning, longer rehabilitation and stress on the cardiovascular system (Edwards 2000). In the *gate control theory of pain*, which since the early 1970s has prevailed in almost every pain-treating health discipline, ascending and descend-ing central nervous system (CNS) processes are thought to filter out, compete with and modulate the neural signals carrying the pain stimulus (Melzak 1999). Con-sidering the analgesic potentials of music and rhythm, Achterberg employed the gate theory, positing that the fast neural messages sent by rhythmic aural input compete successfully with the comparatively sluggish pain messages in the nervous system fibers (Achterberg 1985, p.43). Here is another aspect of music that because of the blending of music and rhythm in DMT may contribute to a potential mechanism for movement's capacity to reduce pain as well.

Melzak recently revised the gate theory to an even more comprehensive and systemic framework called the *neuromatrix theory of pain*. He stated, "the body is perceived as a unity and is identified as the 'self'," and explores the question "How can we explain our experience of the body?" (1999, p. S123). Melzak's "body–self neuromatrix" is "a theoretical framework in which a genetically determined template for the body–self is modulated by the powerful stress system and the cognitive functions of the brain, in addition to the traditional sensory inputs" (p.S125). In Melzak's model, cognitive and sensory dimensions of the pain expe-rience are integrated and interactive with environmental and physiological input (see Figure 4.1).

The theory is remarkably compatible with DMT's goal of integrating physical, cognitive, social and emotional aspects of functioning (American Dance Therapy Association 2002) and contributes to the field for discussion yet another neurophysiological explanation for DMT's effects.

Pain is of clinical concern in chronic problems resulting from injury or surgery, in cancer care, and in stress-related conditions, such as lower back pain (Gallagher *et al.* 1989), with many autoimmune diseases and in the psychogenic somatic disorders. When viewed as a body–self neuromatrix, it is easy to accept the psychosocial and emotional aspects of pain, and to advocate for mind/body interventions in pain treatment programs.

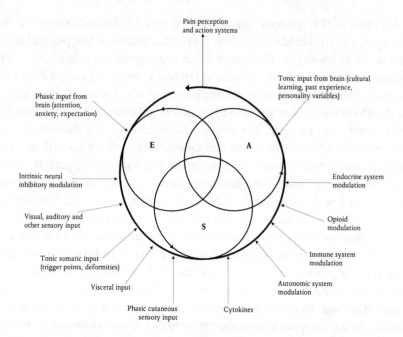

Figure 4.1 The body–self neuromatrix. The body–self neuromatrix, which comprises a widely distributed neural network that includes somatosensory, limbic and thalamacortical components, is schematically depicted as circles containing smaller parallel networks that contribute to the sensory–discriminative (S), affective–motivational (A), and evaluative–cognitive (E) dimensions of pain experience. From Melzak, R. (1999) "From the gate to the neuromatrix" in Pain, 6 *(August), supplement, pp. S121–6. Reproduced with permission of the International Association for the Study of Pain.*

Dance/movement therapists working at the New England Rehabilitation Hospital (NERH) provided a full complement of assessment and therapeutic services to chronic pain and other patients in that physical medicine setting (Ascheim *et al.* 1992). Kierr and Pilus (n.d.) recall the impressive growth and model work of the NERH service team:

> Starting as one movement therapist in a private rehabilitation hospital in Woburn, Massachusetts in 1978…the movement therapy department grew to twelve therapists who worked with physical therapy. Inpatients and outpatients with brain and spinal cord injuries, chronic pain syndrome, and amputations were included in the movement therapy programs. (Kierr and Pilus n.d., p. 1)

Susan Imus, ADTR (personal communication, July 12, 2002; Gorham and Imus 1999), part of the NERH team, drew on psychodynamic developmental theory, humanistic psychology and cognitive-behavioral approaches in later work on the treatment team in the HMO-sponsored Harvard Community Health Plan's Pain Program. Patients were mostly working people who had non-malignant pain for six months or more. They attended between one and three sessions per week for a six- to eight-week program. The program consisted of psychoeducational groups that provided a foundation of understanding. In it patients learned about the biopsychosocial model, basic neurophysiology, and self-care using stress management practices. One goal of the psychoeducational component was to communicate that the health professionals understood the pain and accepted that it is real and "in the body." An initial goal for patients was to accept their pain and stop fighting the body's felt experience. Imus taught creativity theory as a way to approach problem solving, and mind/body theories in relation to creative expression. She also gave instruction in Effort theory (Laban 1980) and about the developmental rhythms of movement (Amighi et al. 1999; Kestenberg 1975). Other dance/movement therapists working with the chronic pain populations also use mainly educational approaches in their sessions (Schalkwijk-Vanderdruk 1993).

The other major component of the Harvard program was experiential, and offered in three different types of groups. The first, which for the purposes of this program was labeled "Dynamic Relaxation," was a standard DMT group conducted in the Chacian approach (i.e., following methods developed by Marian Chace; see Sandel, Chaiklin and Lohn 1993), augmented by the occasional movement homework assignment. For this, a patient may be asked to follow or track movement awareness in a diary or to practice movements independently. This was behavioral work, the goal of which was to find comfort in the body. A second group, labeled "Expressive Relaxation," was multimodal, with art, music, storytelling and laughter therapy. Imus relied on her graduate-level training in art therapy to support the work in these modalities. For the "Aquatic Movement" groups, Imus led Chacian-style movement interaction in the swimming pool.

DMT in an aquatic setting is a variation of the modality suited to the needs of chronic pain patients, and may be considered a "water therapy" (Janco 1991, p.39). Other water therapies are known as hydrotherapy, pool therapy, water exercise, aquatic fitness, aquatic therapy (Janco 1991) or Watsu (an abbreviation of "water" and "shiatsu") (S. Imus, personal communication, July 12, 2002). The DMT variation may involve one person "holding" another in the water, and essentially dancing while supporting release of tension. Imus' sessions also involved deep relaxation and guided imagery, and in them the chronic pain patients at Harvard could gain a sense of flow in their joints. The water provides a sense of buoyancy, and light pressure on the body surface that can feel like a gentle massage (Janco 1991, p.34). In a Master's thesis on the topic, Janco described the dynamic movement qualities elicited in the swimming pool setting. In short, the work facilitated a widening in the body with slow and fluid qualities. Janco also related patients' comments indicating that working in the water reduced pain and anxiety, increased the range of movement, and enhanced mood and social skills. Imus believes that the dance/movement therapists' understanding of movement qualities (i.e. the Efforts) and competence with nonverbal attunement make them well suited for providing water therapies.

In assessments, Imus observed a generalized movement profile for this population: a propensity to move in mobile state, with Effort combinations of the motion factors flow and time. There was often difficulty using *sustained time* and patients needed to learn pacing at the movement level. Tension flow rhythms of the "run–stop–go" type (Amighi *et al.* 1999) predominate. In the water, patients experience the yielding, indulging converse of that rhythm, the "drifting" tension flow rhythm.

In DMT groups, Imus taught patients "slow flow" or, in Laban's Effort terminology, *sustained free flow phrases*. She relates the case of one man, a former boxer, who because of his unremitting pain was suicidal when he entered the program. His very physical background drew him to the movement modality and the therapy began with the structure of tai chi forms. Through the formal patterns of tai chi he initially learned ways to feel in control and manage his pain. Once the clinical relationship was established in movement, the patient could venture into creative improvisation. In this way, he developed free flow in his movement quality repertoire. As the therapy progressed he was able to generalize the mastery of free flow into other activities of his life, and he was no longer suicidal.

In agreement with Kaplan's observation that pain and suffering are distinct experiences, Imus posits that the suffering associated with pain is housed in the patient's relationship to the pain. This is related to the idea of meaning. What is the patient's relationship to the disease? What does it mean to him? While treatment may not be able to "cure" the pain at its source, there can be a revision of that relationship, and less suffering.

Furniss (1998) described Cole's program of group DMT for pain sufferers on an inpatient unit at New England Rehabilitation Hospital (Cole 1988 as cited by Furniss 1998). This three-part treatment sequence built on Jungian and object relations theories, Kübler Ross's stage of adjustment to loss, group theory, and Chace's approach to group DMT, incorporating Bartenieff Fundamentals™ (Bartenieff 1980), tai chi, art and psychodrama methods, circle dances and Bioenergetics (Lowen 1976). In the first of three phases in Cole's program kinesthetic and "here and now" awareness were emphasized. In the second phase, patients worked to accept and embody the body parts and aspects of themselves that had been split off from awareness in an effort to move the salient problems from their somatized state to the emotional expression. Finally, patients worked on how to transfer gains in awareness, expression and relationship to the rest of their lives, by directing newly freed physical and psychic energy into more effective coping with the pain (Furniss 1998, pp.59–61).

Melzak (1999) outlined how hormonal influences in the pain and immune system pathways can render women more susceptible than men to pain syndromes. Research by Wallace (2000) currently underway investigates the effectiveness of DMT for those affected with conditions such as fibromyalgia and reflexive sympathetic dystrophy (RDS). These are both painful disorders with higher incidence in women. Outcome is determined by patient self-report, and this is considered appropriate for measuring a phenomenon that is as subjective as pain.

A Swedish team, Bojner-Horwitz, Theorell and Anderberg (2003), tested changes in self-perception of mobility, life energy and movement pain in women with fibromyalgia who participated in DMT sessions. For this, the researchers employed a randomized two-group design, several hormonal measures, and an assessment technique in which participants viewed themselves moving on videotape. Differences in video ratings by treatment and control group members between baseline and follow-up measurement points suggested benefits in all three aspects of self-perception for those in the treatment group only.

Interventions related to DMT have also shown benefits for pain reduction. For example, Singh et al. (1998) evaluated a pilot program of cognitive-behavioral interventions for fibromyalgia patients. The program included an educational component, relaxation and Qi-gong, an ancient Asian movement discipline, and yielded significant self-reported reductions in pain, sleeplessness and fatigue, with improvements in mood state and general health. Subjects credited the gentle movement sequences of the Qi-gong with providing pain relief and feelings of self-control.

Psychogenic somatic disorders

Sobel (1995) noted that somatic symptoms are "a final common pathway through which medical illness, psychiatric disorders, and emotional distress are expressed" (p.235). Statistics show that "10%–20% of patients presenting in a primary care setting have a diagnosable psychiatric disorder, [yet] more than 80% have evidence of significant psychological distress" (Sobel 1995, p.235). In the overlap between psychiatric disorders and diseases with primary biological etiology are the psychogenic illnesses. Wickramasekera (1998) placed the somatizing disorders on a continuum with psychophysiological problems, and listed the many physical symptoms that *can be* emotionally derived: "chronic fatigue, chronic allergic reactions, chronic pain, muscular and vascular headache, irritable bowel syndrome, temperomandibular joint pain, primary insomnia, low back pain, and primary hypertension" (pp.81–2). In addition, with psychogenic pain there is often a minor mood disturbance "in which the dysphoric mood lowers the thresholds for both pain tolerance and pain perception" (Barker, Burton and Zieve 1982, p.92). Psychogenic somatic disorders and psychogenic pain disorders comprise a class of conditions sometimes categorized as psychosomatic and characterized by the absence of observable physiological cause (Barker *et al.* 1982). The phenomenon is controversial in medical circles because the definition itself implies a culturally bound worldview that separates mind and body. McWhinney, Epstein and Freeman (1997) confronted this assumption in terms of the mind/body integration:

> First, we need to accept that emotions are normally experienced in the body
> …indeed, all symptoms, whatever their origin, have some affective coloring.
> Whether they are experienced as emotions may or may not be abnormal,
> depending on the patient's cultural background. (McWhinney *et al.* 1997,
> p.749)

McWhinney *et al.* (1997) proceeded to suggest a treatment approach, and while they did not refer to DMT, their recommendation is remarkably compatible with the principles and techniques of the modality:

> The connection between emotions and bodily state must be made at the
> affective and cognitive levels by the patients themselves… Physical therapies
> may also be effective in helping patients to make the breakthrough to a new
> level of understanding, without the requirement of verbalization.
> (McWhinney *et al.* 1997, p.749)

Because of the diagnostic challenges they present, these disorders have been called medicine's "unsolved problem" and its "blind spot" (Wickramasekera 1998, p.82). In psychogenic somatic disorders, the underlying or original problem is hidden even from the consciousness of the patient and interventions must be sensitive to the patient's need to defend the psyche from overwhelmingly threatening memories, thoughts or feelings (Wickramasekera 1998).

Lewis Bernstein proposed that dance/movement therapists are capable of this delicate work because they are "aware of and skilled in the interrelationship between psyche and soma, and can facilitate a healing process from both foci simultaneously" (Bernstein 1980, p.45). She presented the case of Celeste, a young woman with rheumatoid arthritis (RA) who experienced her own physical symptoms as connected to emotional and sexual conflicts. The therapy relied on symbols, dreams and fantasy improvisations of the psychic themes. A predominant theme involved the client imagining herself as a princess locked in a castle, and she expressed her experience this way: "It all has to do with each other – my anger, arthritis, sex blocks, cystitis, and the princess" (p.49). Gestalt techniques were integrated into the movement therapy to enable thorough exploration of the body symbols that emerged. For example, in one session the therapist suggested, "Be your arthritis, and let us hear in words what it has to say" (p.47). The therapist also incorporated the use of a private journal for the client, homework and Jungian sand tray work.

Silberman-Deihl and Komisaruk (1985) described a metaphor-based approach to the DMT of somatizing patients, defining bodily metaphor as "a symbolic representation expressed in the form of bodily posture or movement" (p.37). These postures and movements should be understood as nonverbal communication about internal psychic conflicts, feelings and attitudes. In the case of Ted, who had lost his wife to murder, extreme shoulder pain manifested his own murderous and unexpressed rage at his wife's killer. With psychogenic somatic problems there is often a symbolic relationship between the intra- or interpersonal conflict and the body organs or systems affected. The joint pain Ted experienced was linked to the physical act of striking out in anger against the killer. As Pennebaker discovered (Berry and Pennebaker 1993), the constraint of expression about traumatic memories has negative health implications. Silberman-Deihl and Komisaruk reported that "exaggerating and performing the movement revealed the meaning of the pain to the patient...a highly specific body metaphor of the conflict between performing and holding back from performing, a violent act" (p.42). Rossman (2000) relates the case of a priest with severe shoulder pain, who was also restraining the expression of anger. For the priest, the pain was simultaneously a symbol of the internal conflict and a way to avoid addressing it.

In a program for people with psychosomatic disorders at the Karolinska Institute in Sweden, dance/movement therapist Karin Thulin (1997) sees patients suffering from chronic pain and other conditions (including fibromyalgia, headache and RA) for anywhere from 16 sessions to two years of treatment. She observed that many experienced trauma or emotional deprivation in childhood and explained the mind/body dynamic of these conditions in terms of *alexithymia*, or the inability to distinguish and describe one's emotions:

> On a fantasy level, a person who cannot deal with what he/she has experienced by using adequate concepts and symbols, may instead get caught in a

somatic pattern of reaction since other ways of expressing one's emotions are lacking...

One way of helping such people is to use nonverbal techniques to help them see the connection between their current situation and their physical reactions. In this case, creative arts may be an alternative in the treatment of psychosomatic disorders because they are very effective in creating moods and providing symbols for experiences of an emotional nature. (Thulin 1997, p.26)

Working with a woman named Inga who had RA, Thulin first suggested "Try to move inside the limits of your pain," and then facilitated a harmonization of breath and movement patterns. This, observed the therapist, can increase the range of movement available. The psychotherapeutic process unfolded over a two-year period with development of a meaningful, dynamic therapeutic relationship and shifts in the focus of the therapy such that the patient became increasingly able to express both troubling and positive emotions. In the end, Inga reported a higher pain threshold and that she felt stronger, more in control of her life. Thulin observed that as Inga's muscle tension decreased, her joint mobility increased and there was more variety in her qualitative movement dynamics. Thulin clarifies that the chronic medical conditions may well persist, yet pain and muscle tension can be ameliorated and the patients can live with less suffering.

The gastro-intestinal (GI) system is highly responsive to distress and emotions, as demonstrated in the laboratory research on neuropeptides by Pert *et al.* (1985). The skin also expresses psychological conflict and distress (Barker *et al.* 1982). Currently dance/movement therapist Linni Deihl, ADTR, treats patients with a variety of GI conditions including colitis and irritable bowel syndrome, and skin disorders such as eczema. "These are very real medical problems that originate in stress" (Linni Deihl, personal communication, October 7, 2002). Their physicians refer these patients for dance/movement psychotherapy, usually after extensive medical testing has found no physiological reason for the complaints. People may have been struggling with the medical issues for years by the time they begin DMT and are often desperate for relief, ready to explore the mind/body connection that may be the root of their distress. They are monitored medically by their physicians during the course of DMT.

Deihl defines the goals of DMT for this population as somewhat similar to any psychotherapy objectives:

1.   Abatement of physical symptoms.

2.   Acknowledgment of what has occurred in one's life in relation to the health process thus far.

3.   Learning to live with any chronic problems, to cope: some patients' psychogenic conditions have caused permanent damage to their physical bodies. Their therapy focuses on finding ways to live differently.

4.   Problem solving and insight geared toward building healthier relationships.

5.   Improving the sense of self-worth: ego building, identifying strengths, identifying healthy and beautiful parts of themselves and quieting internalized self-deprecating messages from childhood.

The therapeutic technique is a combination of techniques based in the Chacian approach to DMT, Gestalt therapy and methods from Bandler and Grinder's Neuro-Linguistic Programming™ that address kinesthetic experience (Bandler and Grinder 1979). A therapeutic dialogue might begin with the client's simple description of his current state: "I feel tied up in knots." Deihl will start there, with the body-level experience: "I'm not sure what you mean, can you show me how that feels in your body?" The client may then find a posture to represent the tied-up feeling. The therapist will ask, "How tightly are you tied?" and psycho-physical exploration of the experience will be guided by questions and probes such as, "Can you talk about it and show me at the same time?… Can you exaggerate that?… Is there a feeling with this?… Is this familiar?" And when Deihl observes an emotional response, she may ask "How old are you?" This is a developmental approach that invites the client to move the past into the present and to stay involved in the bodily experience. Deihl describes how this helps the client come face to face with the physical sense of the problem and to recognize the area of conflict. Childhood experiences that impinge on functioning can then be reframed from an adult perspective. At this point, the client can see what intrapersonal or interpersonal dynamics may be operating at a level deeper than the immediate life stressors. The premise is that when the client can demonstrate the experience on a physical level, he can integrate his own physical–emotional connection. Deihl emphasizes that the therapy teaches ways to reduce symptoms using the mind/body connection, but does not reinforce the patients' guilt over having created their own medical problems. Rather, the focus is on coping and learning to live with what might be a chronic medical illness.

For patients with skin problems, Deihl works with the role of the skin as a real and metaphoric boundary between the internal experience and the outside world (Montagu 1971). The skin is considered part of the body's defense system (Sherwood 1997) and it is not surprising that this physical boundary becomes a site for the expression of conflicts between the external environment and internal states. Hives, boils and other eruptions are addressed from this standpoint. For example, Deihl may invite a client with skin problems to explore how tension and stress are "held in." Deihl related the case of a successful businessman with severe anxiety and disturbing, recurrent skin eruptions all over his body surface. In the DMT he learned ways of coping, how to deepen his shallow breathing, and to soften his sudden percussive movement style. In addition, he worked directly with his feelings of rage towards his family of origin. Deihl reports that the skin eruptions abated dramatically.

Deihl usually contracts with new psychogenic somatic disorder patients for short-term therapy of six weekly sessions, with homework. At the end of six weeks, closure includes suggestions for self-care, and clients will "try it on their own" for several weeks or longer. They will return every few months for a single session to reconnect with any lost skills, or for a new evaluation. The course of DMT includes homework, and the rationale for this is twofold:

- First, it is a way to cognitively process something that is very experiential, and to continue the work done in session.

- Second, it builds ways for the client to be autonomous in the work.

In brief therapy, it is important to build this component into the therapy from the beginning. Homework assignments may include:

- keeping a diary of feeling states
- noting what one is thinking about right before an attack of symptoms
- noting what is happening right before an attack
- noticing and noting any stressful situation that week, or
- remembering a dream.

Eating disorders of both the restrictive and the overeating types can result in medical problems, and are generally assigned a psychological etiology. However, these problems are generally addressed first as behavioral or psychiatric and later as medical (e.g., when an illness develops secondary to the disordered eating). For the purposes of this text, anorexia nervosa, bulimia nervosa and psychologically motivated overeating are outside the scope of this text. DMT sources on this topic include works by Burn (1987), Hornyak and Baker (1989), Krueger and Schofield (1986), Wise and Kierr Wise (1985) and the aforementioned piece by Silberman-Deihl and Komisaruk (1985).

Heart disease

The psychosocial aspects of heart disease have been well addressed by the field of behavioral medicine. A range of issues have been investigated: from early discussions about the coronary prone Type A personality traits (driven, hostile characteristics) (Seides 1986) to an understanding of loneliness (Lynch 1977) and depression as risk factors, to recent work on the influence of intimate relationships and the role of optimism in successful cardiac rehabilitation (Coyne 2000; Revenson 1994). The heart is not only a vital organ, but also a metaphor for love, caring and emotions. Therefore a malfunctioning heart may have mind/body implications at several levels: psychophysiological, emotional, relational and spiritual. This is a medically heterogenous population, with the term *coronary heart disease* (CHD) serving as an umbrella diagnosis for a number of other physiological events and components. They include:

> Angina is the recurrent chest pain associated with insufficient amounts of oxygen reaching the heart muscle (i.e., ischemia). MI [myocardial infarction] refers to the actual death of a portion of heart muscle (i.e. myocardium) following prolonged ischemia. CAD or coronary artery disease [is] the slow, progressive narrowing of the arteries otherwise supplying blood to the myocardium due to the buildup of fatty deposits on the interior artery walls. (Smith and Nicassio 1995, p.21)

Based on a very few works, there is qualitative and anecdotal evidence that DMT has benefits for patients with heart conditions. Seides (1986) offered a comprehensive rationale for DMT in cardiac rehabilitation work. DMT, she noted, "provides worried, depressed patients with tangible evidence that they can and are expected to regain their physical health and that they will not be hurt by activity" because it "involves movement in a low-key, non-threatening way" (Seides 1986, p.88). Therapeutic foci in Seides' work include the adjustment to a new and realistic body image, sensing the return of vitality, and awareness of inner sensations from the body. "Patients must find a mid-point between fearing and respecting their body signals" (p.90). Cardiac patients need to externalize thought and feelings, and Seides highlights the need to address losses associated with the disease, or the treatment. As shown in Pennebaker's (Berry and Pennebaker 1993) and Krantz's (1994) research, this expression is important to both psychological and physical health. This cardiac DMT program ran weekly for eight weeks, and the significant others (spouses) of heart patients were welcomed. Recalling systems theory, and research on the importance of social support and the strength of the intimate relationships for the health of *both* partners (see Revenson 1994), I see this as a key component of Seides's program. She relates the following lovely vignette about empathy, and the spouse's experience. Imagine a group of about ten people, standing in a circle:

> M. [the wife] put her arms around her husband. "I always feel a need to protect him," she said. "I used to tell him to slow down. After surgery he felt better and could do more, but I still worried about him because I couldn't feel the difference (that he felt) in my own body." M. went on to express her feelings of anxiety when R. [her husband] got sick and her inability to ask for support. "I needed to hold on to my feelings so I could be the supportive one." As M. spoke, individuals moved closer together, eventually standing shoulder to shoulder, supporting M. and one another. There was no need for words. The group had heard and responded on a movement level. (Seides 1986, p.96)

Another application of DMT in cardiac rehabilitation is as a form of stress management. In a group-oriented program reported by Neuman-Bluestein (1999), the DMT uses explorations of personal space and of passivity, education in body and self-awareness, postural alignment techniques, relaxation and creative options for the expression of anger. Participants are equipped to "sense in the moment the cost of a particular stress, which in that moment allows the client options, a key to health and wellness" (p.76). In addition, Hyle (1996) provided an experimental case study of Bartenieff Fundamentals™ (Bartenieff 1980) for a single male patient in cardiac rehabilitation and suggested that the patient's heart rate and blood pressure stabilized with the intervention.

Melsom (1999) presents the brief DMT of a 66-year-old man, a former teacher, who was hospitalized in an acute phase of ischemic heart disease. Therapy focused on the management of unbearable pain due to multiple concurrent conditions (edema, arthritis and diabetes) and unresolved grief after the death of his wife from cancer a year earlier. Working at the bedside, Melsom mobilized not only body action in a warm-up, but also the expression of emotions and imagery that brought the patient to memories of his wife. During the two DMT sessions held during the hospitalization the patient used props (silk scarves and small foam balls) symbolically to communicate sadness over his many losses, learned relaxation techniques, tried new movement patterns that avoided arthritic joint pain, and problem solved around seeking appropriate social support after discharge.

The relaxation response, with its overall inhibition of the sympathetic nervous system (SNS), is beneficial for cardiac patients when part of total stress management programming, particularly for hyypertension, or high blood pressure (Friedman, R. et al. 1996). We know that DMT activity does not bring about the relaxation response but, as Seides proposed, DMT provides moderate exercise in a supportive relational environment, and there may be positive direct effects from this. Schneiderman and McCabe (1989) explain how the CNS responds differently to different kinds of stress, and this may have implications for the use of DMT with heart patients. They summarize the work of Frankenhaeuser (1983) in this way:

> Effort without distress (e.g., exercise; playing a video game) is associated with elevated catecholamines and suppression of cortisol secretion; effort with distress is accompanied by an elevation of both catecholamines and cortisol; and distress without effort (e.g., situations making an individual feel helpless) is associated with elevated cortisol. (Schneiderman and McCabe 1989, p.353)

DMT, offered in the context of a psychoeducational cardiac rehabilitation program and coupled with relaxation work, could provide "effort without distress." This would contribute to the conditioning of the heart while avoiding the cortisol-producing effects of distress.

Pulmonary disease

Diseases of the lung and respiratory system present numerous body/mind issues. Breathing is a sign of living, and difficulties with breathing are often attended by morbid fears. Several such disorders are chronic in nature and are thus amenable to psychosocial support and healing-oriented services. Tapp and Warner (1985) note that biomedical science has achieved control over many of the communicable (infectious) diseases that historically caused most deaths, yet "for chronic/degenerative disorders the biomedical model has been less successful in finding causes and cures ... [and so] different treatment and prevention strategies are called for in dealing with chronic disorders" (Tapp and Warner 1985, p.2). Most of the adult disorders discussed in this chapter can be considered chronic, and cancer is viewed as a chronic disease as well.

Chronic obstructive pulmonary disease (or COPD) is an example of a respiratory disorder requiring a biopsychosocial approach (Kaplan 1990), as are asthma and emphysema. We have evidence that exercise is a valuable component of pulmonary rehabilitation programs for those with COPD (Murphy 1988). Stone and colleagues (1997) have data to show that relaxation can ameliorate the frequency and intensity of asthma symptoms. Using a research technique called "ecological momentary assessment for naturalistic settings," they found that daily use of a relaxation audiotape increased peak expiratory flow rates (the volume of air that can be expelled in a single strong exhalation), which is a clinically relevant measure of lung functioning. In addition, hypnosis has shown benefits for asthma patients, with several studies reporting that patients using hypnosis have been able to reduce their use of medications and bronchodilators (Wagaman 1999). Again, deep relaxation can bring about parasympathetic nervous system dominated bronchoconstriction, and is not always recommended for those with asthma.

To date there are few studies or reports in DMT for adults with primary respiratory illness. Goodill (1995, in press b) conducted a study of DMT for cystic fibrosis adults who were hospitalized with exacerbation of the illness. Cystic fibrosis (CF) is a chronic and life-threatening disease with genetic etiology. It is a multisystem disease involving GI, reproductive and respiratory systems with lung problems constituting the most debilitating and dangerous aspects. The study involved 24 men and women in a randomized, controlled, repeated measures design to test the hypothesis that patients in the treatment group would show more positive mood state, a more positive body image and better adherence to self-care regimens. Treatment group participants received three individual or small group adapted DMT sessions while control group participants received no directed psychosocial support services. Measures included the Profile of Mood States (POMS), the Machover Draw-A-Person (DAP) test and a self-report questionnaire about self-care activities. Mood state and adherence were also assessed in a one-month follow-up. Trends towards better mood state for treatment group participants were evident, but not statistically significant. Compared to those in the control group, treatment group participants reported significantly better adherence to nutrition regimens at the follow-up measurement point one month after discharge from the hospital.

The treatment involved a modified use of group DMT, with a directive leadership style and including relaxation with guided imagery. The goals of the therapy included:

- humanizing the hospitalization experience
- mobilization
- increasing the flow of energy throughout the body
- taking initiative for one's own bodily experiences
- facilitating a positive experience of breathing.

Expressive movement work followed a warm-up that focused on the relief of typically held upper-torso tension, widening of a chronically concave chest region and mobilization of physical energy (see Figure 4.2). Verbal and movement interaction focused on ramifications of the disease on body posture, perceptions by others, expression of feelings about the disease and its treatment, and coping. Relaxation exercises had a strongly kinesthetic focus and the guided imagery was directed towards the process of breathing (see Chapter 9). The sessions were

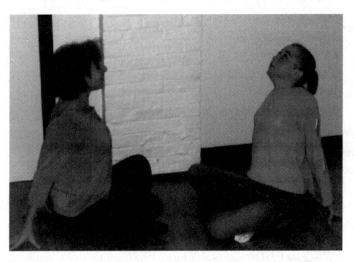

Figure 4.2 A young woman with cystic fibrosis warming up in a dance/movement therapy session. Photograph by E. Goodill. Reproduced with permission.

accompanied by taped music. Within the standard format described above, sessions were tailored to the needs and interests of the patients participating. Some patients came on oxygen or with intravenous (IV) poles and had minor limitations in movement range. Spontaneous responses from subjects in the sessions provide anecdotal evidence for the usefulness of the therapy. During expressive movement interaction, one young man safely used his IV pole as a symbol of his disease and its control over his life. He directed angry gestures towards it and shouted his doctor's name, channeling and discharging the anger that could otherwise become an obstacle to cooperating with treatment regimens. In a discussion among three women after the guided imagery, one woman shared that she uses her own imagery to "get through" the many painful medical procedures: "I just picture my children. I'm doing all this for them."

HIV/AIDS

AIDS (Acquired Immune Deficiency Syndrome) is a progressive disorder for which there is no known cure at present. It is caused by a class of retroviruses collectively and commonly known as HIV (Human Immunodeficiency Virus). People whose blood contains antibodies to HIV are classified as HIV+.

For reasons cited below, HIV is considered a chronic condition:

The human immunodeficiency virus, type 1 (HIV-1), which is a retrovirus of the human T-cell leukemia/lymphoma line, is the causative agent of the acquired immunodeficiency syndrome (AIDS)... Because the potential exists in the HIV spectrum disease for patients to remain free of clinical symptoms for a prolonged period and because appropriate patient management can delay the onset of frank AIDS, it may be useful to view HIV as a chronic disease. (Schneiderman *et al.* 1994, p.267)

There is substantial research on psychosocial services for AIDS patients and their caregivers, including several studies in the psychoneuroimmunology (PNI) field. For reasons not well addressed in the literature, gay men and their partners have comprised most of the study samples reviewed even though more recent epidemi-ological data shows the incidence of HIV/AIDS spectrum disease more evenly distributed across demographic groups. While the usefulness of psychosocial and mind/body services may vary, basic PNI findings may generalize across gender, racial and socio-economic differences.

Kemeny (1994), a research leader in the psychoimmunologic aspects of AIDS, reviewed and summarized studies on the many potential psychosocial influences on viral status in HIV/AIDS. As mentioned above, most of the studies focused on the gay male community. The list of influences below is adapted from her critique:

1.   Psychological hardiness: inconclusive evidence for a positive effect.

2.   Grief: clear evidence for a negative effect when grieving the death of an intimate.

3.   Chronic depression: clear evidence for a negative effect.

4.   A stressful event: inconclusive evidence for a negative effect.

5.   Negative expectancy: clear evidence for a negative effect.

6.   Combinations of other, even inconclusive, negative influences listed above – clear evidence for negative effect.

7.   Psychoactive drugs: no evidence of negative effect.

8.   Group therapy: inconsistent evidence for positive effect.

9.   Aerobics: clear evidence of positive effect.

To this list one must add relaxation, as there is also good evidence for the benefits of programming based on relaxation training. This was reported by Schneiderman and colleagues (1994) in a series of studies with recently notified HIV+ men. Notably, the "frequency of relaxation practice was negatively corre-lated with progression [of disease] ($r = -.71$)" (Schneiderman *et al.* 1994, p.282). The researchers were not able to attribute the benefits to adherence, and wondered "whether the relevant factor is 'conscientiousness' in pursuing health behaviors in general or whether the decreased progression is due to specific aspects of the intervention program" (pp.291–2). Optimism, a sense of personal control, and the ability to derive meaning from the experience all appear to exert an effect opposite to that of negative expectation. Thus, optimism seems to provide a buffering effect against disease progression, especially in the earlier stages of the disease (Taylor *et al.* 2000).

As of this writing, a paucity of published material on HIV/AIDS exists in the DMT literature, and the brief review below is based on Master's thesis projects focusing on psychosocial support.

In Geer's plan for a DMT service program for people with AIDS, he identifies touch as a critical need. He quotes Baer, Holm and LeWitter-Koehler's observation that since "AIDS is a disease of isolation, the importance of touch cannot be emphasized too much. In this illness it is appropriate and often necessary to touch the patients in the course of giving care" (Baer, Holm, and LeWitter-Koehler 1987, as cited in Geer 1990, p.53). Geer emphasized the dance/movement therapist's particular skill with therapeutic interactive touch in the dance/movement context, to "ease the pain of isolation" (p.53).

A handful of DMT Masters' theses have piloted programs for people living with HIV/AIDS and their family members. Comer (1992) provided a description of group DMT for HIV+ gay men. Hartstein (1994) reported positive feedback from participants in two introductory DMT workshops conducted in an urban community setting. Coburn's (1995) case study of a patient with three diagnoses (schizophrenia, HIV+ status and chemical addiction) focused on the patient's capacity for "experiencing" in DMT. Foglietti (1995) conducted four group-DMT sessions with five HIV/AIDS patients and documented improvements in a factor labeled Positive Readiness and Expectancy, as measured by the Herth Hope Scale. Westwood (1995) studied the experience of four men who were living with AIDS and who participated in a 15-week DMT program that culminated in a performance piece. Self-reported quality of life assessments and qualitative analysis of interviews with the men suggested that the modality has potential for catalyzing psychological, physical and social change for this population. Hiller (1996) used videotape analysis to discern the potential benefits of five DMT sessions for men in symptomatic and asymptomatic stages of HIV infection. Hiller's analysis suggested that participants may have experienced social support, emotional expression, self-awareness, reassessment of identity, and exploration of trust, developmental needs and self-esteem issues during the brief course of therapy.

Neurological conditions

Insult to the CNS, whether by injury or disease, can cause global loss of functioning in physical, cognitive, emotional, motoric and social domains. Compared to the work in some medical areas like HIV/AIDS, the DMT literature is rich with clinical description and outcome data in the area of neurorehabilitation. The conditions treated in this context are known as traumatic brain injury (TBI), closed head injury, neurological insult, or simply head injury. For the purposes of this discussion, spinal cord injury is placed into this same category. Berrol and Katz provided a succinct rationale for the role of DMT in neurorehabilitation:

> Movement augments kinesthetic, proprioceptive, tactile and vestibular reception; it completes the feedback loop. These basic sensory-motor functions are crucial to cognitive, physical and emotional reorganization in the aftermath of severe cerebral pathology. It is during this chaotic and vulnerable period that sense of self and understanding of self in relation to the external world are grossly distorted, when confusion and disorientation are markedly manifest; it is a time of behavioral fragmentation. The inherent ability of movement to facilitate and enhance mind–body wholeness provides a powerful tool for lower order nervous system functions and their reintegration with higher order cerebral operations. (Berrol and Katz 1985, p.48)

The authors suggested that in the early phases of neurorehabilitative DMT the therapist should use a directive approach, then gradually the patients should take more initiative and responsibility in sessions. Consistency in format is key (Berrol and Katz 1985, p.51). It is important to incorporate cognitive exercises for memory throughout the therapy, including repetition. This is easily worked into the closure phase of sessions when activities and sequences are reviewed verbally. Movement structures on the themes of passivity and activity address the issue of dependency that can create troublesome obstacles to progress (p.55). Kierr Wise defines the scope of the work in medical rehabilitation with adults this way:

> The movement therapist designs treatment not for strength or dexterity but for personal adjustment. The movement includes elements of work and play. The movement therapist is a member of the medical team and fully able to further the functional goals, like strengthening and dressing. But the movement therapist is not restricted to functional mobility, and can explore movement for the sake of expression and relaxation as well. (1986, para. 26)

Katz's case of a young man, seriously impaired and wheelchair-bound after a car accident, exemplifies how the creative processes intrinsic to DMT facilitated progress (Berrol and Katz 1985). Katz helped him slide from the chair to the floor so he could lengthen, roll and use the tactile feedback from the floor to (a) sense his full alignment and (b) travel through space under his own power and will. As he regained some control of torso positioning and could sit stably, other functioning could be recovered.

Clinicians agree that the use of music in DMT is recommended for this population for the reasons Berrol outlined in her discussion of rhythm (1992) and because of the dynamic of music that can support emotional content. Kierr Wise (1981) saw the potential for music and sound exploration to substitute for movement when the injury prohibits activity. The "music investigation" may ask patients to remember sounds (with both positive and negative associations) and then explore their meaning. Visual images and therapeutic metaphors may evolve from the sound and its stories, or movement functioning may be directly enhanced. Kierr Wise recounted the course of treatment with an accomplished man, a physician paralyzed by metastatic cancer lesions in the thoracic area of his spine. Movement was controlled, and unsatisfactory for him until he discovered the sound of flute music. He associated this music with his son, and released into a more expansive use of his body. Kierr Wise described how his breath "lengthened and deepened… [He] began to use his body and breath to flow from one [modified yoga] posture to another. The lift, stretch, reach, and release became sequential… [and] gave a similar release to his shoulders, back, torso, and hips" (Kierr Wise 1981, pp.49–50).

Musical accompaniment also catalyzed Kierr Wise's therapy of a young woman who, after years in a coma following a tragic pedestrian–car collision, had recovered speech and some motor functioning. Through body empathy, humor and musical associations, the therapist found a way to "join" the patient, Karen, in the important normal adolescent themes of sexuality, rebellion and friendship (Kierr Wise 1986). In this way, Karen could recover some of the psychosocial development that was interrupted when she was struck by the car at age 16.

To recover one's functioning after serious neurotrauma can be an overwhelming process. Kierr and Pilus (n.d.) addressed the need for courage and how DMT can call forth the patient's capacity to confront the daunting task of recovery.

> The choreography of the dance of this therapy is taken from the past, present and future of the injured person. The dance draws comfort from the past and courage from the future. In what way can the future offer courage? Courage appears in positive images: memories of comfort and fantasies of achievement. In dance/movement therapy, patients are guided to access bodily felt memories and the sense of well being that gave them feelings of safety, power and control in their pasts. Then they begin to risk moving in their present,

with the injuries their bodies have sustained, drawing on the positive tools
uncovered from earlier challenges in their lives. (Kierr and Pilus n.d., p.2)

A handful of case studies have yielded encouraging but limited results. Guthrie
(1999) used a mixed-methodology, experimental single-case design and a nine-
week course of daily individual DMT sessions for a 30-year-old man injured in an
auto accident. Guthrie documented clear responses to treatment in the domains of
movement quality (Effort elements) and movement control, using video analysis
and the subject's self-report, and concluded that there was a cause-and-effect relationship between the DMT and the movement changes observed. Dijkwel (1998)
conducted a multiple case study of group DMT for five head injured patients in a
six-week course of treatment (twice weekly sessions of 30 minutes each). Progress
was evaluated through self-report and with the Functional Assessment of Movement and Perception (FAMP: Berrol *et al.* 1996; Berrol *et al.* 1997). With mixed
results, the researcher concluded that measurable progress was contingent upon
the frequency of attendance in the groups, and the patient's perception of the
therapy. The patients who attended at least ten sessions and enjoyed the groups
showed gains ranging from 24 to 28 per cent on the FAMP.

In what is arguably the strongest single clinical outcome study conducted to
date in the field of DMT, Berrol and colleagues (1997) investigated the effectiveness of group DMT for elders who had sustained non-progressive neurological
insult (e.g. stroke, TBI, cerebral aneurysm) (see also Berrol *et al.* 1996). In a
well-controlled pre-test–post-test design with both quantitative and qualitative
measures, the researchers studied the domains of physical functioning, cognitive
functioning, mood and social interaction. Conducted in multiple sites with
multiple therapists, the study included 134 (after attrition 107) subjects of diverse
cultural/ethnic backgrounds. Measures included the FAMP, the National Institute
on Aging Frailty in Injuries Cooperative Studies Intervention Techniques Battery,
the Cognitive Performance Scale, the Geriatric Depression Scale, the Multidimensional Observation Scale for Elderly Subjects and an adaptation of the
Minimal Data Set. Subjects in the treatment group(s) received 45-minute group
DMT sessions twice weekly for five months, and the control subjects received
standard care that did not include DMT. At post-test, the treatment group showed
significantly more positive change on several variables, when compared to the
treatment group. Specifically, these were in cognitive performance (decision
making, the ability to make oneself understood and short-term memory), social
interaction (self-initiation, ease with others and activities, goal setting, accepting
invitations to join others and involvement in group activities) and three items on
the FAMP (the backwards walk, sideways walk, and a range-of-motion reaching
task) (Berrol *et al.* 1997, pp.145–6). Qualitative data from subject questionnaires,

video analysis of sessions and therapist reports concurred with the qualitative results. The study constitutes a compelling demonstration of DMT's effectiveness with this population.

Normal aging processes have their own health complications, including a gradual weakening of the immune system (Sherwood 1997), but aging itself is not a medical condition. Nonetheless, there are some neurological conditions usually diagnosed in old age that are considered primarily medical. Parkinson's disease and Alzeimer's disease are two such disorders, and dance/movement therapists have explored a role for the modality in their treatment and management.

In a well-conceived study of how DMT may benefit Parkinson's disease patients, Kaplan Westbrook and McKibben (1989) compared the effects of six weekly DMT group sessions to those of six weekly exercise groups (the control condition) in a crossover design (N=37). Dependent variables included depression, as measured by the Beck Depression Inventory (BDI), and walking time (number of seconds to walk 32 feet). Movement impairments dominate Parkinson's disease and *bradykinesia*, or difficulty initiating movement, is the most debilitating symptom (Kaplan Westbrook and McKibben 1989, p.29). Thus, the walking time parameter represented the fluidity and ease with which the subject could initiate locomotion and travel through space, and was used as an indicator of neurological and functional status. A paired t-test analysis of group means showed significant differences between treatment and control conditions in walking time, with shorter walking times at the DMT post-test measurement. Changes in BDI scores were insignificant.

Certified movement analyst and dance professor Janet Hamburg has developed a successful movement program, "Motivating Moves"[C], for Parkinson's patients (Parkinson's Disease Foundation 2004). It is based in Laban Movement Analysis (LMA) principles (Bartenieff 1980), and designed to improve several functional and dynamic aspects of movement. In related work, a variation on the Motivating Moves[C] program was found to improve balance and gait characteristics in a study cohort of 36 healthy elders (Hamburg and Clair 2003).

A large observational study of dementia risk in the elderly (Verghese *et al.* 2003) found that dancing was associated with lower risk of dementia, and dancing was the only one of nine physical activities examined to show this relationship. Writing on the topic of DMT and dementia care, Hill (2003) stated, "The art of dance is about structure (through rhythm and shape), and about involvement and focus" (p. 264). These features of the art form, which integrate cognitive and motor domains, might shed light on the Verghese team's findings and could make DMT a potential treatment of choice for elderly people with encroaching or established cognitive decline. Earlier, Hill (1999) reported on a phenomenological

study of brief DMT for an 85-year-old woman with dementia (presumably Alzheimer's). The therapist/researcher incorporated videotaping, so that the subject
watched her own DMT sessions. This would facilitate memory, and allow the
patient to integrate visual information about her own body and movement experiences. Self-awareness and reminiscence were supported and enhanced, evidenced
by the subject's own perceptions: "I've got together again... I've always been
tough... Thank you for bringing me out of my shell" (Hill 1999, pp.16–17).

Child patients

The developmental context

Any psychosocial assessment or services to children or adolescents with medical
illness, whether chronic, acute or life-threatening, needs to take into account the
child's developmental levels, the systems in which the child lives, and individual
characteristics of the child or adolescent (La Greca and Stone 1985). This basic
premise of clinical behavioral pediatrics, also known as pediatric psychology, is in
keeping with the systems and biopsychosocial theories presented in Chapter 1.
Engel (1980) proposed a hierarchical chain of systems operating in his biopsychosocial model. Engel's model for the "interactional nature of systems" (Engel 1980,
p.537) begins with the individual person (including experience and behavior) at
the center of the chain, and then follows the interconnections between systems
within the individual's progress into smaller and smaller units to the level of
subatomic particles. Interconnections between systems external to the individual
are shown to progress in larger and larger units as far as the level of the biosphere.
For practical purposes, when providing psychosocial care to medical patients, the
range of systems in our attention might span from Engel's cultural–subcultural
level to the nervous system level.

When the ill person is a child, the role of the family system, the child's care-
takers, becomes essential to health and survival. Elaborating on systems theory
specifically for pediatric psychology, Kazak (1989) drew on the work of
Bronfenbrenner (1979) to outline a social–ecological framework for this work.
The concept is easy to grasp using the image of concentric circles, as follows:

> Social ecology is defined as the study of the relation between the developing
> human being and the settings and contexts in which the person is actively
> involved. The model proposes that the child is at the center of a series of con-
> centric circles, which represent settings that have bidirectional influences on
> the child. The concentric rings that are further away from the child are those
> that represent societal values and culture, whereas those closer to the child

indicate settings of a smaller scale, such as family, neighborhood, and school. (Kazak 1989, para. 8)

Psychosocial, emotional, cognitive and pscyhomotor developmental assessment is already part of the Master's level dance/movement therapist's repertoire of skills. To this one must add an understanding of how the child's developmental functioning shapes his or her experience of illness, hospitalization and treatment. Kazak (1989) further recommends the evaluation of parents, siblings, extended family and support networks. In each stage of development, different issues are salient. The discussion to follow is a composite of material contributed by Bibace and Walsh (1980), La Greca and Stone (1985) and Prugh (1983).

The guiding question is "how do children's conceptions of health and illness change as a function of changes in their developmental status?" Six developmentally ordered categories of explanation (i.e., the child's explanations for the illness) have been articulated. These categories are consistent with Piaget's three major stages of cognitive development (Bibace and Walsh 1978). In the pre-operational stage, the phenomenon of the illness is defined by a single external and obvious symptom. The child's idea of how disease is acquired is based on contagion, where the source of the illness may be imagined as a person or object spatially near to, but not touching the ill person: "You just catch it." Illness may happen as consequence of bad behavior or even for magical reasons (La Greca and Stone 1985). In the concrete operations stage, the child distinguishes between what is internal and what is external to the body. The child understands that illness is inside the body, and that illness can be reversed. A cause-and-effect perspective has developed: one gets a cold from "germs in the air; you breathe them in," or people get cancer "from smoking without their mother's permission" (Bibace and Walsh 1980, p.292). A child in the formal operations stage will consider multiple possibilities for the disease: organ malfunction, personal actions and psychological contributions, and can accept some degree of ambiguity about causation. There is an understanding of some simple disease processes and this can bring about a sense of control.

The emotional experience of illness and hospitalization presented by Prugh (1983) rests on Erickson's theoretical framework of development. Infants and toddlers are mastering developmental tasks concerning the establishment of trust and subsequently, autonomy. These children will manifest behavioral and psychophysiological reactions that are consistent with separation anxiety, and the separation itself may have as much of an impact as do the medical procedures and actual illness. For preschoolers, responses to the stressors and separations involved in hospitalization include regressive behaviors, and the disturbing sequential pattern of "protest, despair and detachment" (Prugh 1983, p.503). Older preschool children, who are developing a sense of initiative and have a sense of their body's integrity, will experience fear of pain and bodily mutilation. Emotional themes for school-aged children undergoing medical procedures will involve the fear of loss of control over what is happening to their body and fear of harm to their body. The experience threatens the sense of industry that children of this age are mastering. Adolescents will usually fear the loss of newly acquired independence. It is normal for teens to react emotionally to the ways that illness will impact on their personal identity and sense of future, that are by now valued and part of their consciousness. The identity is linked to the peer group, and the loss of that social support is a psycho-emotional threat as well.

Throughout childhood, social maturity is a factor in the child's adaptation to illness or hospitalization. La Greca and Stone (1985) present the issues from a social development perspective. In the preschool years, the family is the child's social world and relationships with parents are critical. Thus, the separation issues that characterize this phase have social implications as well. The seriously or chronically ill grade-school child may miss a good deal of school, and thereby miss opportunities for developing friendships, early peer group experiences and the social skills that are built in these contexts. As mentioned above, teens in this situation may look and often feel "different," which is *socially* difficult. To gain a sense of belonging in the increasingly important peer groups, teens may adopt behaviors that are dramatically more risky than for their healthy peers: smoking, drinking, etc. Non-adherence to the medical self-care regimens is another way to assert one's independence and try to fit in, but this is clearly maladaptive and dangerous for teens with chronic illness.

In addition to these domains, the dance/movement therapist considers the development of the child's body image, which is a multidimensional process involving kinetic, proprioceptive, tactile, neurological, cognitive and social input (Schilder 1950). With illness, pain, disfigurement, surgery or invasive procedures, the developing child's attention and emotional energies are redirected to the affected body parts and zones, altering the formation of the body image accordingly (Goodill and Morningstar 1993). Pylvänäinen (2003) proposed three properties of body image that are relevant to DMT and this discussion:

- body memories (that are held in the body and the mind)
- felt experiences (that are sensed and felt in the present moment) and
- imagery (visual aspects of the image, how the body is "seen" by the brain and mind).

Assessment may access information about all three, but DMT treatment methods are likely to impact the second property, felt experiences. Mendelsohn (1999) advised that DMT assessment of ill children should try to determine the source of any observable movement deficits, specifically if the child is "suffering from a purely physical dysfunction or weakness, or...from emotional stress and anxiety" (p.70). Cohen and Walco (1999) describe the use of LMA in pediatric movement assessment, and this objective approach to observing subtle qualitative changes in movement should enable the therapist to make the determination that Mendelsohn recommends. If possible, it is best to observe a child over time so changing levels of vitality and body involvement can be put in context. Mendelsohn suggests that appropriate behavioral criteria for referral to DMT, particularly in the inpatient setting, include observed body tension, immobility that is not the result of medical devices or sedation, restlessness or lethargy. Any health care professional can be alert to these qualities. The dance/movement therapists who work with medically ill children incorporate all of these areas into their assessment and treatment procedures, as will be seen in the examples below.

Pediatric medical DMT is practiced across a wide spectrum of health care settings, from the pediatric intensive care unit (PICU) to the inpatient units to outpatient work. This review will include examples of each. As with the disorders affecting adults, the following disorders of childhood and adolescence will be considered primarily psychiatric or behavioral and will not be included in this review: ADD/ADHD, mental disability and problems of disordered eating. Oncology and hematology applications will be discussed in a separate chapter. Medical science has made it possible for children with serious illness to live longer and more normally. Therefore, similar to the adult populations, chronic illness has become a major focus of pediatric psychology (La Greca and Stone 1985) and this seems to be the case with much of the pediatric medical DMT reported to date.

In pediatric medical applications, DMT may aim to:

1.   decrease anxiety connected to hospitalization and procedures

2.   aid in the adjustment to temporary and permanent changes in the body and in functional abilities, and to affirm the positive aspects of the body image

3.   provide an active rather than passive experience with one's body

4.   provide an environment in which feelings about the illness and/or hospitalization can be appropriately expressed

5.   address the total child rather than focusing on disease or dysfunction alone (Goodill and Morningstar 1993).

To these, Mendelsohn (1999) adds the following goals:

6.   to keep alive the movement impulse; to arouse and motivate

7.   to encourage play, out of a relaxed state, to communicate emotional
        pain while preserving necessary defenses.

DMT programming and case vignettes

Irmgard Bartenieff conducted early movement therapy in pediatric hospital
settings, using her combined training in physical therapy and LMA. She told of
work with a group of boys who were confined to their beds for up to two years
with an orthopedic condition that caused deterioration of their hipbones. Her
greatest concerns were for the youngest children who, in the concrete operations
stage of cognitive development, still needed physical activity in order to learn and
integrate experiences, and "it became apparent that cutting off the possibilities of
movement was like cutting off life itself" (Bartenieff 1980, p.7). Bartenieff
developed a movement program that emphasized Effort dynamics and mobilized
the boys even while in bed, including dancing with props that they themselves
had fashioned.

In the outpatient Pediatric Pain Program of UCLA Children's Hospital, DMT
Nicholas Kasovac observed that by the time children presented to the specialized
program, they would have endured multiple diagnostic tests, undergone many
invasive and painful procedures, and encountered dozens of health care practitioners (N. Kasovac, personal communication, August 9, 2002). They entered the
program looking anxious, psychologically defended and frightened, expecting
that more physical contact would cause more pain. Kasovac, who is also a licensed
massage therapist, gave these children massage, integrating DMT skills based in
LMA and Kestenberg Movement Profile (KMP: Amighi et al. 1999) concepts.
With modulation of the weight Effort towards sensitive, delicate qualities of
touch, and careful adjustment in spatial relationships (planes of space and shaping
dynamics), the movement communication inherent in a massage therapy session
created a safe psychological and physical environment.

For some children, dance/movement was the treatment modality of choice.
Kasovac relates the following case study (personal communication, August 9,
2002). Bethany was a nine-year-old girl who suffered from migraine headaches
and fibromyalgia. She was very involved in gymnastics and dancing, and was dis-
couraged that her ailments kept her away from the activities she loved. DMT
assessment showed a predominance of muscle tension and bound flow, especially
in the areas of her neck, shoulders and chest. She could not yield her body weight
and appeared stiff and tight. Kasovac's work first focused on the stiff, bound flow
by teaching her to use a passive release of her body weight and free flow
movement phrases. Using the physioball, she practiced risk taking, balancing,

rolling and softening to fall. Later she started to use dance improvisations, assuming the role of a dancer and displaying the abstract movement patterns that she imagined a dancer might use. There was an emphasis on positions, and on movement "tricks." The therapist encouraged more expressive, creative aspects of movement and from there he guided her into breathwork, helping her access feelings using vocalizations and sounds. Bethany became able to relax the neck–chest–shoulder area. As she and her parents perceived the incremental improvements in her movement flow and body comfort, returning to her physical activities became her main goal. She did meet that goal and went back to gymnastics and dancing.

This case demonstrates the roles of imagery and expectation in health, as presented in Chapter 2. When Bethany improvised like a dancer, it was as though she was imagining herself out of her painful, constricted condition. She was envisioning and, more important, mobilizing an image of herself as a pain-free and healthy girl. Second, we see the role of hope, expectation and belief. When Bethany started therapy, the pain and impairments were great and the goal of returning to full functioning may have been more depressing than motivating. However, after a little improvement, some possibilities and hope emerged. She had the usual minor setbacks during the course of therapy, but her progress was steady and focused. Her parents communicated their belief in her ability to get better, acting as part of her health care system and reinforcing her fledgling sense of self-efficacy. Kasovac notes that Bethany's pain conditions were attributed in part to conflicted family dynamics, as is true for many of the children presenting chronic pain problems. This makes it all the more significant that Bethany's parents found a way to support her recovery.

Josephs and Kasovac (1999) recommended the following for DMT with chronic pain disordered children:

Movement reduces the learning process about the body to basic, fundamental levels, much like babies learn in a sensorimotor fashion. Let children start there.

1.   Don't focus on the pain itself. Give lots of play and let the child experience pleasure as a distraction.

2.   Teach breath control and increase breath capacity.

3.   Give the child control over what happens in the session.

4.   Include some yoga: when holding positions, muscles can tire and fatigue. It is possible then to release stubborn tension that causes pain.

5.   Expand expressive range. This leads to an expanded perception of options for individual functioning.

Children can also present with psychogenic somatic disorders, and ocassionally as victims of the factitious disorder, Munchausen's-by-proxy. More common are the children who present with chronic pain as in the case of Bethany, or another medically inexplicable syndrome. These children are often manifesting family conflict or stress, and might be diagnosed with conversion disorder or "somatic disorder" (Susan Imus, personal communication, July 12, 2002).

Imus describes the illustrative case of a seven-year-old boy who had had a chronic cough for several months. While he was away at camp, his mother was in an auto accident and was hospitalized. The boy first developed anxiety and then the cough, which persisted long after the mother had returned home and recovered. By the time the family came to the pain clinic, a pediatrician and a family therapist had tried unsuccessfully to determine the cause. In two sessions, using creative expressive techniques (movement, metaphor, art, storytelling) the dance/movement therapist was able to elicit the beliefs and fears behind the symptom. The boy thought that his mother was going to die, and no one in the family had imagined he harbored such ideas. In this case, the DMT functioned primarily to clarify diagnosis in a difficult case. However, the therapeutic value to the boy of disclosing his somatized fears should not be underestimated.

Dance/movement therapist Pat Mowry Rutter (personal communication, July 18, 2002) encountered another psychogenic condition in the child populations she treated at National Jewish Medical Center in Denver: vocal chord disorders. This problem mimics asthma, but is normally less severe, and there are psychological issues involved. The tightening of the vocal chords can feel like the beginning of an asthma attack and there is a great deal of fear with that sensation. Mowry Rutter provided breath interventions in the form of yoga breathing exercises, so the children could learn to work with the constriction using the exercises themselves. This augmented the speech therapy, which was the primary therapeutic modality for children with this disorder.

Asthma, the most common pediatric respiratory disorder, affects 5.5 million children in the U.S., and incidence of childhood death from asthma is increasing. Illustrating Kazak's assertion that socio-economic and cultural systems play a role in child health, the death rate is higher among African-American children than in any other single ethnic group (statistics from the Asthma and Allergy Foundation of America 2002). Severity can range from mild, where the child is inconvenienced by occasional wheezing and the need for self-administered bronchodilators, to frequent attacks of wheezing that are debilitating and require intensive medical attention. An asthma attack can be life threatening and is quite frightening to the child and anyone witnessing the attack.

The children seen in the asthma program at National Jewish Medical Center in Denver generally have serious illness. This is a specialized multidisciplinary program for children aged one month to 20 years old. Mowry Rutter (personal communication, July 18, 2002) and an art therapist provided milieu therapy to children and teens. This work is described below. Overall goals for DMT with the asthma population included:

1. Adherence. It is vital that asthmatic children and their parents find ways to manage the illness without imposing on the psychosocial development of the child, nor infusing the household with conflict and stress over the issue of adherence. Most psychosocial services make this a priority for asthma patients (Lehrer, Sargunaraj and Hochron 1992).

2. Facilitate good parent–child communication. This leads to better adherence, and more normal development.

3. Address issues of bodily trauma. As with other chronically ill pediatric groups, the accumulated trauma of multiple invasive procedures leaves its imprint on the body image as well as on the physical body.

4. Either decrease extremely overcautious living, which evolves in response to medical traumas like tests and resuscitation, and an overall sense of one's fragility; or decrease the recklessness that appears in asthmatic children who are in denial. Children who fling their bodies through space and let themselves crash and be hurt need to become more attentive to their bodies, to "feel themselves" in a physically sensitive way.

5. Learn to recognize and modulate, channel and express emotions. Mowry Rutter observed that emotions would often provoke an asthma episode.

Mowry Rutter saw that if the children and their parents could truly engage in the psychosocial aspect of the program, the children showed more medical improvement. A family focus was critical to the success of the psychosocial program. The parents of younger children were often included in the DMT. Mowry Rutter observed that the separation process was often disturbed in the asthma families. Parents raising a child who can unpredictably go into an asthma crisis can become overprotective, and understandably so. The relationship can look enmeshed, too close. Conversely, as the child attempts to reject the many restrictions imposed by the disease and the parent who enforces them, the relationship can become detached. In parent/child DMT, Mowry Rutter would structure mirroring activities (with the child or the parent "leading" the other in movement) and see either merged or disconnected interaction patterns. One child would mirror his mother exactly, in total attunement; another would not let himself reflect his mother's movement. Struggles over adherence to medical regimens were often underneath a child's defensive refusals to "join" with a parent in this activity, and the therapist would help the dyad explore the movement pattern in relation to that issue.

In addition, Mowry Rutter taught yogic breathing with visualization to parents and children alike, and some would practice those exercises at home. Sometimes Mowry Rutter would see just the parents in a DMT session and sometimes the family as a whole.

DMT assessment of the population suggests two predominant body attitudes in asthmatic children.[1]

1. A bulging flared thoracic area. This is an anatomic phenomenon. The ribs can become "flared" after years of using auxiliary muscles in that area to support breathing, and from the almost constant retention of stale air in the lungs, that become too weak to make full exhalations.

2. Concavity in the chest area. This can be seen as emotionally driven, perhaps to draw inwards and "protect" the vulnerable area of the body.

Complex motivations and maladaptive reactions can play a role in childhood asthma as well. Mendelsohn (1999) describes a DMT session with an asthmatic boy hospitalized after a severe attack. The playful movement interaction with the therapist unearthed a dynamic wherein the boy confided that he used the illness to avoid feelings of inadequacy as well as the task of confronting his own feelings. He disclosed, for example, that for health reasons he had to take the school bus when his friends could walk, and this was embarrassing to him. This was short-term DMT, and following the disclosure Mendelsohn referred the family to appropriate outpatient mental health services.

Severely asthmatic adolescents struggle with a host of body image and social issues. After years of maintenance on steroid medications, these children develop a bloated, "moonfaced" appearance. Metabolism and appetite are also altered by high dose steroid treatment. Consequently, these teens are often overweight.

---

1   Kestenberg (1975) defined body attitude as "the way the body is shaped, how it is aligned in space, how body parts are positioned in relation to one another and to the favored positions of the whole body. It also denotes all the patterns and phrases of movement for which there is readiness at rest. In addition, it indicates the qualities of movement which, through frequent use, have left their imprint on the body" (p.236).

Osteoporosis, another side effect of the steroids, causes back problems that can require wearing a back brace. It is no surprise that adherence is a problem in this subpopulation. Experiencing the social stigma of these disease sequelae, the teens found the DMT support groups at National Jewish Hospital a place to belong and relax. "They would find it a relief to be together" and the group became close, honest and supportive (Mowry Rutter, personal communication July, 18, 2002). Themes of anger and body control prevailed in the group of adolescents. For example, from rhythmic group movement a strong pattern would emerge. This could mobilize and channel anger in a safe form of group expression. The group would set a sequence, master it and repeat it until it was exact, then make a small dance piece from it. Games with props that required balance, communication and teamwork embodied the theme of gaining control, and the teens would be proud of these fun and physical accomplishments.

A multiple case study of DMT with asthmatic children (Barlow 1983) incorporated the clinical technique of "breathing together" (Blau and Siegel 1978), where the therapist places her hand on the child's chest and the child's hand on hers, then using eye contact and verbal coaching the two establish matched breath rhythms. This is a format for teaching new breathing patterns. The five subjects, children aged between seven and eleven years old, all showed increases in peak expiratory flow rate (PERF), a clinically relevant measure of pulmonary status.

Loughlin (1993) describes a successful DMT program in Australia for adolescent girls and women who have Turner's Syndrome, a chromosomal disorder that affects the endocrine system and commonly results in short stature, abnormal pubertal development and infertility. The goal of the program was to address the attendant psychosocial issues of the syndrome. Although Loughlin's program included grown women, the work is reviewed in this section because medical and psychosocial difficulties emerge in childhood and adolescence. Throughout their lives, girls and women with Turner's may experience social isolation and troubles with assertiveness, a sense of inadequacy associated with their infertility, and the body image issues that build up in teens who look and feel "different." Along with the older women, the teens in Loughlin's groups were seeking an experience with others who knew their plight. Consistent with the lack of assertiveness and a lifetime of feeling socially "invisible", the DMT participants had difficulty activating the weight Effort in movement (Loughlin 1993, p.118). This dynamic movement quality is associated with sensing one's physical presence, intention, verticality and the use of force (North 1972). In the DMT groups, which ran for four years, the girls and women responded well to structured group improvisations using "strong, formed shapes" (Loughlin 1993, p.116), props that supported clear shapemaking (big cushions, bamboo sticks, ropes, blankets and baskets) and musical accompaniment with strong melodic and orchestral features. The outcomes of the therapy were entirely psychosocial, with attention to support and coping. Loughlin observed evidence of progress when group members reported making changes and taking action in their communities and careers, and in direct positive feedback about the DMT.

Mendelsohn (1999) proposes that pediatric medical DMT is concerned with three levels of movement phenomena: the body/functional level, the interpersonal level and the symbolic level. At the symbolic level, "the child engages in creative play through which he or she expresses fears and wishes or unconscious thoughts" (p.74). Imagery and creative play characterized the DMT on an inpatient pediatric unit reported by Goodill and Morningstar (1993). Two preteen girls with chronic illness, one with epilepsy and one with cystic fibrosis, used movement symbolism in their small group DMT session to reinforce a feminine identity and express hope in their own futures. With a bedsheet for a prop they actively imagined swimming in the ocean, and growing from seeds into tulips and trees. Using pantomime, they "sculpted" imaginary gifts in the air and gave them to each other and the therapist. Their gifts to the therapist, make-up and jewelry, were "in keeping with their view of her as a grown woman, but may also be seen as a view of themselves as women" and a symbolic statement of their intent to grow up (Goodill and Morningstar 1993, p.26).

A DMT perspective can support ancillary medical care even in a highly technological environment. Kasovac reports work in the Pediatric Intensive Care Unit (PICU) of the UCLA Children's Hospital with very young children who had serious liver disease (personal communication, August 9, 2002). Serious congenital conditions such as biliary atresia (failure of the biliary system to develop) may result in liver failure by the age of about three years. Kasovac would observe these children following organ transplantation, when they would spend months at a time in the PICU. Children have nascent verbal skills at this phase of life, and so a focus on nonverbal communication enables the treating adults to perceive their emotional state and their needs. Kasovac found that training in LMA and the Kestenberg Movement Profile (KMP: Amighi et al. 1999) enabled accurate, effective observation of how the children were coping with their disease process, medical interventions, the intensive care environment, their families under stress, recovery after surgery, and other variables in their experience. Kasovac and Loman (1997) presented a case study of DMT for an infant who developed cardio-myopathy (damage to the heart muscle) following a non-progressive myopathy (muscle weakness), and required a heart transplant. Using the KMP as a pre- and post-test measure, several improvements in psychomotor functioning were noted, including more balance and greater organization of qualities across the profile, and more Efforts were available (Kasovac, personal communication, October 4, 2002). These changes can be interpreted as enhancement of the baby's resources for coping with the stressed internal environment (after surgery) and the demanding external environment (of the hospital setting).

Through these observations Kasovac has derived an interesting hypothesis regarding body image formation in these young, technology-dependent children. They have lived much of their short lives attached to medical devices such as gastrostomy tubes for feeding, central line catheters, or ventilators. These ever-present devices sustain life and breach the body's natural boundaries to do so. The younger children (aged between one and two years) wouldn't understand that the machines are part of their survival, but older ones (between three and five years old) generally did. Regardless of the level of cognitive development, the children are aware that anything done to the machine is directly affecting them, and they appear to relate to the devices as an extension of the body. The machinery seems to become grafted into the internal representation of the body and incorporated into the body image. This notion is worth exploring further in mind/body research with very young children in these circumstances.

Medical status is the primary concern for critically ill children in the PICU. However, there is still a need to relieve distress when possible, and Kasovac would give massage to these bed-bound children. Weaning a child (or anyone) off a ventilator requires evidence that the child can succeed at breathing alone. For some children in poor pulmonary status, the immobility itself mitigates against the regaining of strength for independent breathing. To support the weaning process, Kasovac would provide gentle, specific massage to the torso region to stimulate circulation and muscle tone. Some children were maintained under sedation on high frequency, low volume ventilators in order not to overwhelm fragile lungs. Even touch was contraindicated for children in this weak condition, so Kasovac learned and provided therapeutic touch interventions. In therapeutic touch the practitioner uses his or her hands to mobilize the patient's energy field without physical contact and requiring no conscious participation by the patient (Ireland and Olson 2000, p.57).

Kasovac's clinical work is an example of a therapist adapting his clinical repertoire to meet the needs of his patients. By extending DMT training and principles to therapeutic massage and therapeutic touch modalities for immobilized child patients, he can provide a full continuum of non-invasive mind/body services as a single practitioner. Wherever the level of medical impairment, the child can then receive some form of non-pharmacological intervention that is appropriate to the child's sensory and motoric capacities at the time.

Therapeutic touch and massage have both shown evidence for effectiveness with pediatric populations. Ireland and Olson (2000) reviewed and summarized the research on both modalities. Much of the best massage therapy research has been conducted by Tiffany Field and her colleagues at the University of Miami. Their studies have shown impressive psychological and physiological benefits for children with asthma (improved PEFR and affect, decreased anxiety), cystic fibrosis (improved mood, anxiety and PEFR), atopic dermatitis (decreased anxiety, improved affect and skin status) and juvenile rheumatoid arthritis (decreased anxiety, stiffness and pain) (Ireland and Olson 2000, pp.58–9). Therapeutic touch (TT) has been explored in qualitative and quantitative research designs, with mixed results and some methodological problems. One study of TT with HIV+ children suggests the method was successful in reducing anxiety (Ireland 1998, as cited in Ireland and Olson 2000) and the reviewers suggest that TT research proceed using more controlled and longitudinal designs.

Pediatric medical rehabilitation is long-term care for children who need residential and intensive medical attention. A subset of children in medical rehabilitation have multiple overlapping conditions with impairment of development and functioning in several domains. This was the case for an eight-year-old boy who received individual DMT with Pat Mowry Rutter over a three-year period (Mowry Rutter, personal communication, July 18, 2002). This case illustrates the capacity of the nonverbal dance/movement approach for teaching relationship skills and helping even the most limited children derive some enjoyment from their bodies. The boy, whom I shall call Thomas, was an unusually fragile child from a medical standpoint. He was born with Down's Syndrome and an immune system disorder, and suffered massive cerebral hemorrhages at birth. At the age of eight, he presented as autistic and hyperactive, with failure to thrive syndrome, hypersensitivity to touch, and no verbal language – only screaming. A cardiac pacemaker implantation, a nasogastric feeding tube and a PIC line (for delivery of immune system medications directly to the bloodstream) all impinged on his movement range. Other problems included head-banging and generally wild, uncontrolled behavior. Most professionals who knew him thought he was inaccessible and unworkable, and found it impossible to "reach" him. His adoptive mother, a nurse, could manage his needs at home for much of the time and so Mowry Rutter saw Thomas in inpatient, outpatient and private venues.

Working with Thomas as one would an infant, the therapist used mirroring techniques and presented numerous balls as props for initiating interaction. Very gradually, she shaped a simple yet playful reciprocal interaction pattern with Thomas. Over the first two years of DMT, formatted in weekly 30-minute sessions, Thomas learned early developmental games: "peekaboo", chasing the ball together, and cuing the therapist with eye contact for the activities he like the best (e.g., being pulled about on a small mattress). The therapist became able to interrupt head-banging episodes with a close, tactile face-to-face intervention. From this interaction, Thomas became able to enjoy different kinds of touch inter-actions with her. He enjoyed short dancing "duets" to classical music, when they faced each other and held hands. He watched baseball on TV at home, and brought into the DMT a "sliding into base" movement game. A personality emerged, and over time Thomas acquired four spoken words that he used in the DMT sessions. Later, his mother stated that no other therapy was able to help him as much as the DMT did. Two years into therapy, at the age of ten, Thomas's func-tioning peaked at an 18-month-old's level.

After this, he went into a medical decline with more head colds, more surgeries and needing a cast on one leg. Previously clear and organized movement patterns became fragmented and diffuse. When cardiac failure set in and Thomas's body became bloated from fluid retention, he could hardly move. Mowry Rutter observed that he was weaker and "fading." Yet in his last DMT session Thomas inexplicably revived old patterns from the therapy. Like an "instant replay" of the previous two years, Thomas reached out to the therapist, made rhythmic, commu-nicative sounds and let himself be held. He seemed less dull that day and displayed some of his favorite movement phrases. The therapist observed some joy, and she sensed that he wanted to keep going. It was as though Thomas was remembering, and wanted the therapist to remember with him – a life review process at the sensorimotor level. The therapist and the mother both had an intuitive sense that perhaps his death was near. Indeed, he passed away one week later.

From this remarkable and unique case we learn two important things. First, Thomas's replay of what he did over two years of DMT suggests that learning went on. With very little capacity for movement or communication, he demon-strated memory and an investment in the therapeutic relationship. We also see how the human life force that motivates movement, Laban's antrieb or "impulse to move" (Laban 1980), can be healthy even when the physical body is failing. Thomas's decline was medical, but his psyche (a term derived from the ancient Greek word for "soul"), stayed active and connected to his small but vital social world of the therapy.

The reader will note that much of the medical DMT reviewed in these pages incorporates one or more other mind/body methods: relaxation, yoga, breathwork, meditation, imagery. Many practitioners include homework in the medical DMT programming as well. These seem to be two ways that conventional DMT techniques are modified and augmented for work with primarily medically ill people.

Some of the variation in approach, goals and structure reported here could be due to different stages and types of illness and disease in clinical populations. As Spira (1997) so coherently outlined, newly diagnosed people need medical education, stress/pain management and social–emotional support more than psycho-educational training or exploration of personality issues. Later, when in treatment, it is important to add a focus on coping skills to psychosocial work, and when in recovery, coping becomes most appropriate. People with chronic severe illnesses such as AIDS or recurrent cancer most need social–emotional support and work focused on moderating stress, pain and mood. Those who have recovered from illness do benefit from depth work and a focus on personality (Spira 1997).

Basic DMT clinical methods are inherently flexible: reflecting and responding to patients' movement initiations, amplifying and clarifying expressions, bringing the sensed and unspoken kinesthetic experience to awareness and facilitating problem solving through creative exploration of movement options. Movement is ubiquitous and present as long as life persists. These features of the modality permit its application across the lifespan, across stages of illness and recovery, and even in the dying process, as will be seen in the chapters to follow.

CHAPTER 5

Dance/Movement Therapy in Cancer Care

This chapter describes the author's own and others' work in various cancer-related applications. This chapter first introduces psychosocial issues in cancer care and provides a broad psychooncology perspective in relation to dance/movement therapy (DMT). The two psychooncology specializations that have seen the most development, DMT for breast cancer survivors and DMT in pediatric oncology, are then covered in more depth.

Dance/movement therapy and general psychooncology

Cancer is not a single disease, but a class of conditions including hundreds of site-specific diseases. All cancer is characterized by a "proliferation of cells that do not contribute to the functioning of the organism as a whole and that displaces cells that do" (Blaney 1985, p.533). The surveillance theory of cancer suggests that the mutation of a normal cell into an abnormal cancerous cell occurs frequently but the immune system, especially the T-cell system, usually detects and destroys such cells. Thus, the proliferation of cancerous cells and growth of tumors, including the spread or metastasis of cancer to secondary sites in the body, is considered a failure of the immune system in its surveillance, "search and destroy" function (Sherwood 1997).

Blaney (1985) reviewed the research on psychosocial aspects of adult cancers available at the time. On the whole there is very little consensus on either the role of predisposing psychological factors or the role of stress in the etiology of cancer. More recent data from psychoneuroimmunology (PNI) studies, particularly the findings that stress compromises NK cell activity, support the notion that stress is a risk factor for cancer (Hall and O'Grady 1991; Irwin *et al.* 1990; Keller *et al.* 1994). Consequently, early attention to predisposing personality factors has by and large been supplanted by research foci on (a) the psychosocial impact of a cancer diagnosis and the treatment process and (b) psychosocial interventions to reduce distress and help people cope while living with cancer. Towards this end, a number of psychosocial interventions have been tested, with outcome variables ranging from transient improvements such as mood state, to behavioral changes, attitudes and coping patterns, to disease progression and survival. This chapter will review some of these studies before turning to DMT interventions in general cancer care. Blaney observed that "there is clearly room for new psychological applications in dealing with the emotional and physical distress of cancer... although it remains to be shown what patients are benefited by what interventions and why" (1985, p.557). Self-help and support groups for cancer patients emerged in the U.S. as early as the 1940s (Benioff and Vinogradov 1993). As of the mid-1990s, cancer patients in most urban and suburban areas of the U.S. generally have access to some sort of professional psychosocial support. This may be offered through the treating hospital, through patient advocacy community agencies or societies, wholistic and complementary health centers, or through organizations like the Wellness Community (Benjamin 1987) that specialize in meeting the psychosocial needs of cancer patients and their loved ones. The emergence of DMT as a psychooncology intervention brings us closer to identifying how DMT might fit into the array of psychosocial options available to cancer patients.

Fawzy and Fawzy (1994) are widely recognized in the health psychology literature for their study of a psychosocial intervention for patients with malignant melanoma (Dienstfrey 2001). Malignant melanoma is a skin cancer, and the leading cause of death among all skin diseases (Isselbacher *et al.* 1980). In the six-week intervention, groups of seven to ten patients met weekly for 1½ hours of health education, stress management modalities, coping skills and psychological support. The stress management component included relaxation, guided imagery and self-hypnosis.

The psychological support component of the program rests on Fawzy and Fawzy's useful model of life's trajectory and the assumptive world (1994, p.372; see Figure 5.1). The assumptive world is a composition of one's life, including the phases and experiences in one's past, as well as one's plans for the future. We are, the authors wrote, on a "life trajectory" (Fawzy and Fawzy 1994, p.372) and a life-threatening illness interrupts that trajectory in radical ways. During and after treatment, cancer survivors live in a new assumptive world. It is a task of the psychosocial health provider to help the patient construct that new, "and possibly better" assumptive world so that he or she can resume their forward life trajectory, albeit changed by the profound experience of the disease (p.373). The conceptualization was built with adults in mind, but children imagine their futures, and so the idea may apply to serious childhood illness as well.

Life trajectory

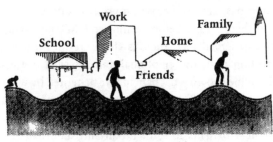

Assumptive world

Life threatening disease

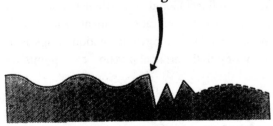

Medical and psychiatric
treatment

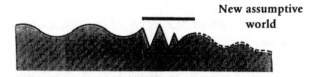

Figure 5.1 Life trajectory model. From Fawzy, F. I. and Fawzy, N. N. (1997) "Psychoeducational interventions and health outcomes," in R. Glaser and J. M. Kiecolt-Glaser (eds) Handbook of Human Stress and Immunity, *San Diego, CA: Academic Press. Reproduced with permission.*

Outcome measures assessed change in psychological and behavioral factors (mood and coping), and immune system activity (natural killer or NK cells) in the patients with malignant melanoma. Measurements were conducted at baseline, immediate post-intervention and at six-month follow-up points. Data were analyzed in a repeated measures analysis of covariance model (Fawzy and Fawzy 1994, p.378). What follows is a dramatically truncated summary of their extensive and impressive findings.

When compared with the control group participants, those who received the intervention showed moderately greater gains in mood state post-intervention, but by the six-month follow-up these gains had increased significantly in magnitude and range. Treatment group participants used significantly more active–behavioral coping strategies at post-intervention, and by six months were also using significantly more active–cognitive coping strategies than were control group participants. These strategies contrast with the less effective avoidant strategies (see Chapter 2 for definitions and discussion of coping). For all immune system variables, the treatment group showed significantly larger benefits. These positive effects were also sustained at follow-up. The researchers established positive correlations between anxiety, depression and poor coping strategies, and diminished NK cell activity. Interestingly, they found positive correlations between higher levels of anger and NK activity.

It is important to note that the researchers viewed anger as "an expression of assertiveness and defiance rather than irritability and rage" (Fawzy and Fawzy 1994, p.387). This is consistent with an expressive therapies framework in which the expression of emotions is encouraged as a productive manifestation of inner reality (Chodorow 1995). It is also consistent with Pennebaker's findings (Berry and Pennebaker 1993) regarding the health benefits of emotional expression, regardless of positive or negative affective valence. Benioff and Vinogradov (1993) related Yalom and Greaves' distinction between justified anger – which can be vented and then mobilized with adaptive coping strategies – and misdirected or irrational anger (1977, as cited in Benioff and Vinogradov 1993). According to the authors, cancer patients experiencing the latter need supported expression and guidance to build an understanding of the anger and the attendant existential issues.

In a randomized controlled study, Baider and colleagues at the Hadassah University Hospital in Jerusalem tested the effectiveness of a brief intervention based on relaxation (Baider et al. 2001). The six-week program included body warm-ups with easy physical exercise, relaxation with guided imagery (a different script and theme each week) and homework. Participants were men and women recently diagnosed with localized (no metastases) cancer. This ambitious study measured change over a three-month baseline period and again six months after the intervention was completed. Patients in the treatment group showed small but significantly greater improvements on the Global Severity Index, a measure of psychological distress. Patients who were more distressed at baseline derived greater benefit, leading the researchers to suggest that future studies screen newly diagnosed patients and offer the intervention only to those who report higher levels of distress. The Baider group's study is relevant to medical DMT because it combined physical activity with psychologically meaningful imagery. Inasmuch as DMT research has suggested its usefulness for short-term state change, it would have been useful for comparison purposes if the Baider team had also collected immediate post-test data at the end of the six-week intervention.

Hypnosis is another mind/body approach used in oncology care primarily for relief from anxiety, pain reduction, and to reduce the nausea often induced by radiation and chemotherapies. Levitan (1999) advises that hypnosis practitioners make their first assessment inquiries about the patient's level of comfort, rather than pain or nausea. This creates the suggestion of a goal or objective, rather than an initial focus on the problem. Levitan's suggestion echoes positive psychology theory and the concept of self-efficacy. It also underscores the importance of language when communicating about the body's experience. This is applicable to medical DMT as well as hypnosis and other mind/body practices.

Anna Halprin describes herself as a choreographer, dancer, teacher and leader of movement, and not a therapist (Halprin, in Serlin 1996a). Her dance/movement workshops with cancer survivors began in 1980 at the Cancer Support and Education Center, California. Her descriptions of these sessions tell of powerful, life-affirming experiences (Halprin 2000) and are relevant to the topic of DMT in cancer care (Seibel 2001). Each of Halprin's "classes" are structured with a verbal check-in opening, followed by sensory awareness exercises (an induction phase) and movement exploration (much like a DMT group warm-up). She then provides thematic improvisational movement structures to guide the participant's creation of a dance. Movement development, expression and sharing are then followed by an art response or private journaling, and the class concludes with sharing and discussion, and a movement closure sequence. The level of structure in Halprin's thematic exercises represents a departure from the conventional practice of DMT, where the patient's spontaneous material provides the content of a session (Sandel 1993b), but Halprin stays observant and sensitive to the needs of her group participants, and she easily revises workshops as needed. Halprin sees dance as healing – she emphasizes ritual, imagery and symbolism, spiritual elements, and a connection to the natural world.

Rider's (1995) MA thesis is a comprehensive review of theory and clinical work related to cancer and DMT. She describes psychooncology work by therapist Fran Ascheim at the New England Rehabilitation Hospital (NERH). Ascheim provided DMT to patients with very little full body movement capacity. Clinical goals included pain management, fostering effective coping, emotional expression, relaxation and stress reduction with a focus on "reinforcing the health intact parts of the self, as well as enhancing the patient's capacity for self-acceptance, self-nurturance and self-expression" (Ascheim, as cited in Rider 1995, p.85). In addition, the program aimed to "restore a sense of control over one's life and body,…maintain hope and motivation for involvement in the present" (Ascheim et al. 1992, p.19). Ascheim's program progressed in stages, beginning with the alleviation of physical discomfort, moving to awareness of internal (emotional) responses, and then to the exploration and release of emotions connected to the illness experience. For the first stages, Ascheim used primarily relaxation and breathing methods, then empathic techniques (Sandel 1993a) to support the emotional expression in movement (Rider 1995).

Dieterich's program (1990) used a technique based on the imagery research by Achterberg and Simonton (Achterberg and Lawlis 1978; also see Chapter 2). After leading participants through the visualization of immune cells, cancer cells and their action, and after making artwork to depict the mental imagery, Dieterich guided her patients into an embodiment of the imagery. They used props (such as pillows and soft bats called batacas), vocalizations and group interaction to express in movement the dynamics of the cancer imagery. Dieterich reports that the women experienced this activity as cathartic and liberating (pp.93–6).

In another individual session recorded on videotape and in written transcript, Dieterich offers her patient a Buddy Band (a large, closed loop of elastic, stretchy fabric), and the act of stretching and pulling becomes a metaphor for survival. As the stretch band lengthens, the patient says, "…I'm gonna' stretch this life as long as I wanna' live… And stretch my days, stretch my years, stretch my life…as long as I wanna' live, and live it well" (Dieterich 1990, p.106; videotape).

In Petrone's study of a six-week DMT support group for adult cancer patients and their partners/caregivers (1997), sessions included warm-up, structured theme development and closure components, as well as work with breath and guided imagery. The participants' journal entries describe the program's benefits, especially for the reduction of isolation, support for expression of feelings and improved attitudes towards the illness. The following samples are from cancer patients who were in treatment at the time, and those who had completed treatment.

This dance/movement therapy lets you know that you are still a part of society. That just because you are ill there are things you can still do and be a whole person, even with your illness.

It [DMT] showed me that I can be more open to others, even people outside of our group.

This experience also seems to break the ice when new people attend the meetings because they will participate in these activities even if they are not ready to talk about their problems.

Dance/movement therapy is more of a physical nature than any other therapy and it is a more distinctive way of expressing what you are trying to say to the group.

Out of doing movement therapy, I received a clear-cut picture of my position in being ill and through recovery... It puts things in a better perspective.

The group movement therapy is a help in overall disposition and outlook on life. [It] takes you out of self-centeredness.

It makes me feel closer to the group and brings a sense of lightness to a very heavy, serious illness.

(Petrone 1997, pp.52–3)

In day-long workshops for cancer patients, I have offered a "journey" exercise. For this, "journey" is understood as a metaphor for life's passages, changes, processes and for how we live through time and space (Goodill 1992). The exercise is a guided movement improvisation in which the mover creates a nonverbal narrative of his or her own, reflecting on a process of growth or change. It is most appropriate for groups of people who are already focused on a shared type of challenge, such as recovery from substance addiction, or from child abuse. What follows is a cursory description of the technique.

The mover begins at one end of the available space and names the starting point in terms of his or her own personal journey. For some cancer patients, this may be the time of diagnosis, or perhaps even earlier in their lives. The opposite end of the available space represents the end point of the journey, however the mover wants to perceive that and label it. For many cancer patients, survivorhood is that goal. With the therapist in a witnessing role, participants travel along a sagittal, forward–back spatial dimension from the beginning point towards the end point, exploring the movement metaphor. For novice movers, this exploration relies on the familiar and movement-rich language commonly associated with advancing and retreating, and with journeying or traveling through one's life.

Examples are: I took two steps forward and one step back... I had no idea where I was going... I was going around in circles... I got stuck in that problem and couldn't get out of it... I fell down and picked myself back up again... and so on. The improvisation is done alone and quietly, but in the company of others. Movers are directed to end their traveling at whatever point in space represents the present moment, and how far they feel they've come on their chosen journey. Afterwards, people are free to share verbally about the content or the process of their journey improvisations.

Two vignettes illustrate the potential usefulness of this method for people coping with cancer. Ruth was a woman her late 60s who had had colon cancer and recently undergone a mastectomy for breast cancer. She had lost her husband to a brain tumor one year earlier. For her, the stress of her own illness was compounded by her continuing and deep grief over the loss of her husband. She was frequently tearful and anxious when describing her present situation. She began her journey exercise with good memories of the beginning of their marriage. She remembered herself as a happy, young bride and her movement was light and resilient in quality, with swaying hips. During this creative and mobile reverie, she re-experienced herself as healthy and whole, and briefly had some relief from the emotionally painful realities of her current life.

At one point in her journey, Sally, a breast cancer survivor in her 50s, stopped and simply fell over forward from the waist. After a moment of stillness, one elbow and then the other lifted at 90-degree angles. From her elbows she became erect again, took a big breath and soon proceeded forward. Later she shared how this sequence symbolized when the cancer came, and how others helped pick her up to move forward again. Later, she wrote, "I feel empowered with a sense of my own body and senses and being able to know what I want to express." It is suggested that the journey exercise is an embodiment of Fawzy and Fawzy's (1994) concept of the life trajectory. This DMT method is an experiential form of reflection and creative re-envisioning of one's life. It may provide a way for cancer patients to develop their new assumptive world.

Recent psychooncology research in DMT includes a study underway in Germany. Researcher and dance/movement therapist Elana Mannheim is investigating DMT as part of multidisciplinary programming, and measuring quality of life as an outcome factor (Mannheim 2000).

Dance/movement therapy for women with breast cancer

There is a substantial body of research on psychological interventions for women who are living with breast cancer. In the last 15 years, virtually every mental and wholistic health discipline in the U.S. has addressed the needs of this clinical population. This section briefly reviews selected studies of psychosocial support interventions using primarily verbal modalities, and then focuses on the growing DMT research literature. For breast cancer and other oncology patients, the need for psychosocial support does not stop with the end of medical treatment, and many programs offer services to patients for an extended time after medical treatment is completed. Physician, researcher and breast cancer survivor Elizabeth McKinley expressed this need when she wrote, "I'm done, according to the medical profession. But I don't feel done. I think we survivors are never truly done. We just move from the quantifiable, treatable disease to the immeasurable uncertainty of survivorhood" (McKinley 2000, p.479).

A 1981 study by David Spiegel and his colleagues demonstrated how group psychotherapy for women with metastatic breast cancer improved psychological well-being (Spiegel et al. 1981). The year-long intervention program consisted of verbal group therapy sessions that met weekly for 90 minutes. This has been described as supportive–expressive group therapy with an existential basis (Serlin et al. 2000). The focus of the therapy was on "living as fully as possible, improving communication with family members and doctors, facing and mastering fears about death and dying, and controlling pain and other symptoms" (Spiegel et al. 1989, p.889). The authors emphasize that they did not include cancer-related guided imagery in the intervention, although patients did practice self-hypnosis for pain control. In a 1992 televised interview with host Bill Moyers, Spiegel described hypnosis as "a state of focused concentration," a combination of mental alertness and physical relaxation, and a way to increase the sense of control (Moyers 1993, p.158). Spiegel asserted the rationale for going beyond the usual support group approach and for providing true psychotherapy. These patients need to grieve and explore issues of death and dying, he said. This requires "focused attention" and "being able to tolerate the very strong feelings that arise when people have to give up their ability to do things" (Moyers 1993, p.161).

Open-membership support groups are quite common and offered in diverse venues and formats. A survey of 131 participants in one such program gathered data regarding frequency of attendance, reasons for attending and the respondents' perceptions of benefits (Pilisuk et al. 1997). This was a YWCA-sponsored program that included a swimming pool exercise component followed by a conventional verbal support group meeting that included educational information and occasional guest presenters, with supportive and informal sharing. The exercise program focused on physical rehabilitation, especially for the arm and shoulder region, and most women felt it was "a vital supplement to recovery," helping them to regain strength and flexibility (Pilisuk *et al.* 1997, p.78). Of interest from a mind/body and body image perspective is the fact that group members of the YWCA program would shower and change clothes in the locker room together between the pool session and the support group. This seems to have been a positive phenomenon: 78 per cent of survey respondents agreed strongly or somewhat that sharing dressing areas helped them feel more comfortable with the changes in their own bodies. The researchers' summary emphasized universality as the primary therapeutic factor. "The discussion session offered a time for women to know that they were not alone emotionally, and the public dressing areas allowed them to realize that others were going through the same experience physically" (Pilisuk *et al.* 1997, p.79).

One study has differentiated the effects of group support and guided imagery with metastatic breast cancer patients (Richardson *et al.* 1997). Two different six-week interventions, a structured support group and imagery sessions, were compared to a standard (medical) care control group. Outcome measures included mood state, perception of quality of life, coping strategies and immune system functioning. Compared to the control group, women in both intervention groups reported enhanced meaning in life and more improvement in coping skills, particularly with more use of support seeking. Women in the support group reported better acceptance of death than did control group participants. When compared with women in the support groups, those in the imagery group reported more vigor, less stress and more quality of life improvement in social and functional domains. Neither intervention influenced immune system functioning.

The question of effects on disease recurrence and survival remains unsettled. In 1989, Spiegel's group (Spiegel *et al.* 1989), conducted a ten-year follow-up with the participants in their original study, and learned that patients from the intervention groups lived an average of 1½ years longer, or twice as long, compared to their control group counterparts (i.e., a mean of 36.6 months from study entry to death in the intervention group compared to a mean of 19.8 months in the control group) (Spiegel *et al.* 1989, p.889). Potential mechanisms for the survival effect included the pathways of influence for social support, the expression of emotions, and better adherence to treatment regimens, possibly including more consistent use of self-hypnosis for pain control. This astounding finding spurred several attempts at replication with metastatic breast cancer patients (e.g., Goodwin *et al.* 2001), and other oncology patients as well (e.g., Fawzy and Fawzy

1994). Results have been mixed and Spiegel recently discussed the state of affairs, noting that in all studies where there was a survival benefit to group therapy, there were also measurable emotional benefits. This is logical, as "a psychological intervention that does not help emotionally is not likely to provide physical benefit" (Spiegel 2001, p.1768). Spiegel's informed assessment is that the psychosocial benefit of supportive group therapy for cancer patients is sufficiently established and the treatment can be confidently prescribed for this purpose, if not for prolongation of life. He recommended that future psychosocial research focus on "identifying the populations that are most likely to need and respond to emotional support" (p.1768). Relevant to Spiegel's recommendation, the Goodwin *et al.* study (2001) uncovered a relevant relationship with regards to psychosocial benefits: that women who reported more distressed mood and more pain at baseline reported more improvement on these variables.

DMT findings on the effectiveness of the modality for women with breast cancer coalesce into the notion that this modality may be particularly beneficial for this cancer population. Anecdotal, descriptive and quantitative data from specialist interviews, Master's projects, doctoral dissertations and published studies are included in this review of DMT for women with breast cancer.

Dance/movement therapist and clinical psychologist Dibbel-Hope (2000) investigated whether DMT could help women with breast cancer increase their level of psychological adaptation to the disease and to the treatment. Thirty-three women, all of whom completed medical treatments 6 to 60 months prior to the study, were randomized into treatment groups (N = 22) or a wait list control group (N = 11). Study participants ranged in age from 35 to 80 years and most (81%) had undergone a modified radical mastectomy as the primary treatment. The intervention consisted of a six-week DMT group conducted in the Authentic Movement format (see Pallaro 1999), with weekly sessions of three hours' duration. Sessions were structured with a verbal check-in; movement improvisations in various group, dyadic, triadic or solo formations; guided discussions of the movement experiences; and a therapist-led movement closure. Outcome variables included mood state, body image, self-concept and levels of distress. Data were collected through standardized self-report psychosocial instruments, semi-structured interviews and subjects' written evaluations. Measurements were taken at pre-test, post-intervention and at the end of a three-week follow-up phase.

Treatment group participants showed significantly greater improvements in three parameters associated with physical well-being: increases in vigor, reduction of fatigue, and reduction of somatization. Interview data suggested that overall, the women in the treatment group found the experience valuable, with 63 per cent identifying social support as a main benefit. All reported an increased awareness and appreciation of their own strength, sensitivity, knowledge and/or hope, and attributed the change to the Authentic Movement groups. Also 27 per cent reported an appreciation of their bodies and 18 per cent felt more accepting of their bodies "as is" (Dibbel-Hope 2000, p.63). Further analysis of the data using stepwise multiple regression procedures led Dibbel-Hope to suggest that DMT delivered in the Authentic Movement format may be most useful for older women, those diagnosed with earlier stage disease, those who had less invasive treatment, those with more time elapsed since medical treatment and those with more past experience in physical activities (Dibbel-Hope 2000, p.60). However, younger women with prior experience in dance and sports reported more positive body image post-treatment. Curiously, there was also an effect of geography, with participants in one part of the state (California) reporting more positive responses. The multiple interacting variables and the study's sample size combine to render the findings tentative (p.64). However, inasmuch as this study has identified specific benefits for a subgroup of breast cancer survivors, it is responsive to Spiegel's research challenge. With this information, dance/movement therapists can begin to target the therapy to women who are likely to derive the most from the treatment.

Dance/movement therapist Joanna Groebel, MA, provided a course of group DMT to post-mastectomy breast cancer patients in a multidisciplinary program with the physical therapy (PT) department at Reading Hospital, Pennsylvania. The PT goals focused on the recovery of musculoskeletal system functioning, and the prevention or reduction of lymphedema. Lymphedema is a painful and incapacitating swelling of the lymph nodes in the arms, which is a common complication following breast surgery. The DMT program emphasized personal expression and body image integration (J. Groebel, personal communication, August 2001), and it became the centerpiece of the hospital's public media efforts to promote its services to women with breast cancer.

A substantial research project is currently underway at the MidState Behavioral Health System in Connecticut, funded by the Connecticut Department of Public Health. Dance/movement therapist Susan Sandel, PhD, ADTR, is providing the treatment in this randomized, controlled study investigating the effectiveness of the Focus on Health through Movement and Dance™ program for women who have undergone surgery for breast cancer (Judge et al. 2002). The Focus on Healing program was developed out of a physical therapy framework in the 1980s by Davis (2002), and in this variation is aimed at reduction of lymphedema and recovery of flexibility using dance sequences. The intervention is quasi-standardized, including the choreographed Focus on Healing patterns and Sandel's DMT-based group interactive experiences. In case of missed sessions, participants can work at home with a videotape produced by Davis. All study participants receive 18 group sessions over 12 weeks, and serve as their own controls during another 12-week no-treatment phase. Outcome variables include range of motion and severity of lymphedema, measured by physical examination; and quality of life and psychosocial functioning, as measured by a battery of self-report instruments. The study team reported initial anecdotal evidence of psychosocial and functional improvements (Judge *et al.* 2002).

The work by dance/movement therapist and psychologist Ilene Serlin, conducted through the California Pacific Medical Center, is exemplary as an integrated, multidisciplinary clinical and research program. The program consisted of 12 weekly sessions, based in an existential approach to group DMT using a form known as Kinaesthetic Imagining (Serlin 1999b; Serlin *et al.* 2000). Healing imagery, healthy sexuality, self-empowerment and relationships are all valued and encouraged in the groups, which employ ritual, meditation, movement expression, play, musical accompaniment, art expression and discussion. In a video documentary of the program (Serlin 2001), psychiatrist Elizabeth Targ underscores the uniqueness and value of the DMT approach in psychooncology. Noting that several mind/body modalities employ visual imagery she observes that "not everybody is visual" in their sensory preferences, and so a body-based, kinesthetically oriented approach reaches some patients who are not helped by the visualization interventions.

Like the expressive–supportive therapy groups used by her colleagues at Stanford, Serlin's DMT groups enable participants to "struggle genuinely" with the existential issues of freedom, death, isolation and meaning (or meaninglessness) (Serlin *et al.* 2000, p.130). Serlin has asserted the essential nature of a process-oriented approach to the group therapy, arguing that as people move towards the goals of a more internal locus of control and more spontaneous self-expression, they need not be simply compliant with a leader's instructions (Serlin 1999a; Serlin *et al.* 2000). The theme of freedom is articulated eloquently in the body sensitive language of a participant in Serlin's groups:

> It gives spaciousness to my cells so it allows them to breathe and allows them to flow more freely and then it gives spaciousness to my spirit because all of a sudden I'm free and joy or pain or whatever comes out… And again, that's where the healing is – is that we don't have to be anything. We can just become who we are and who we're meant to be. (Serlin *et al.* 2000, p.131)

The DMT program unfolds in three phases (Serlin 1999a). First, the focus is on helping the participants learn that they can take time for themselves for their own emotional healing. Next, is the "working" phase, for the authentic exploration of feelings and the struggle with existential issues through creative processes and group sharing. The third and final stage is about mobilizing the gains in one's life and in the community, often with advocacy and activism in the fight against breast cancer (such as fundraising or participation in public events).

Serlin's groups were conducted as part of a multicomponent research project. Body image was a central outcome variable, but existing assessment tools for body image were standardized on other populations and found to be inadequate for measuring the changes achieved in this type of therapy (Serlin *et al.* 2000). Working with colleagues at Stanford University School of Medicine, Serlin has developed a clinically relevant outcome instrument that was derived from movement study and DMT principles (Serlin 1999b). Beginning with qualitative phenomenological methods, depth interviews and videotape analysis, Serlin discerned the critical mind/body themes for the women with breast cancer who participated in the DMT groups. She captured the essence of their bodily-felt experience by retaining their own language in the items comprising the assessment tool, called the Kinaesthetic Imagery Profile (KIP). The KIP also includes a movement observation component that consists of movement parameters based in Laban Movement Analysis (LMA). Serlin (1999b) reported that preliminary movement assessment data from the study pilot suggest trends towards concavity in the torso and a restriction of pelvic mobility in many breast cancer survivors. Research on the validity and reliability of the two-pronged instrument is in progress (Serlin, personal communication, September 2001). The authors aim to produce "a body image scale which is unique to the experiences of women with breast cancer, which can show significant change over time in descriptions and observations that are connected intimately to their own words and narratives..." (Serlin *et al.* 2000, p.131).

This author conducted an eight-week DMT-based support group for women with breast cancer, under the auspices of a Wellness Community. The Wellness Community is a national network of support centers for people with cancer and their families, founded in 1982 by Harold Benjamin with a "Patient Active" philosophy (Benjamin 1987). The Patient Active view embraces the mind/body unity, values communication and community and encourages proactive, mobile participation in the fight against cancer. At the national level, the Wellness Community conducts provider trainings, research and advocacy. At the local level, communities offer a full palette of educational programming. Support groups are the backbone of the Wellness Community's programming but there are also humor groups, mind/body services (such as yoga, tai chi, meditation, visualization work and DMT), bereavement counseling, special workshops, guest speakers, fundraising events and Kids' Circle groups.

My groups for women with breast cancer were open to those in medical treatment and those who had completed treatment. The self-selected participants ranged from 35 to 70 years of age. Weekly sessions of two hours' duration roughly followed Serlin's model with discussion, interactive movement experiences based on themes of support, healing and recovery, and private responses using artwork or journaling. In addition, this program included relaxation with guided imagery exercises. The importance of social support emerged often, in various ways.

During a partnering exercise, people shared weight and explored active and passive support. This took the form of sitting back to back and leaning into one another, or one person shifting to bear the torso weight of the other. In another variation, one partner cradled the forearm or leg or head of another, and the passive partner yielded their weight to that support. The task involved release of tension and nonverbal communication through touch. There was sensitivity to the side where surgery had happened and gentle talk between partners during this time. Later the idea of "teaching husbands to do this" came up, suggesting the need for gentle, tactile support in the marital relationship as well.

In the final session, women were asked to think of a stressor they had success-fully dealt with: "something you have already come through in the process," and to develop an expressive movement pattern that "represents and embodies that challenge." Next, they were asked to develop a movement phrase depicting "how you got through" or coped with the challenge, and finally to creatively combine these two phrases into a "coping dance." Each woman shared her dance with the group, narrating her movement as the others learned it and moved with her. One woman, Bess, began with a sustained bilateral spreading motion of the arms beginning at the site of her surgery. She said, "I came from my breast, lost my breast, it went away, and I am coming out of myself." As she explored the second phrase, she directed the spreading around the circle and brought the movement back to her center. During this she spoke about the groups and how much she had gotten from them. Sue, who was heavily involved the treatment process, had just received her first chemotherapy treatment following mastectomy. She was seeking ways to get through her current challenge, and the movement task brought her attention to two resources. Exploring the movement, she recalled some artwork she owned but had not yet unpacked after moving from out of the area. In it, a woman is shown with her arms reaching. As Sue stretched up and out with both arms she said she was "reaching, and then reaching further." Her second phrase was a long self-hug, squeezing, releasing and squeezing again. She said this repre-sented all of the support and love from others, brought close to her self even though some of her support system lived very far away. She left that day intending to go home, unpack the reaching picture and hang it up to inspire her through the rest of the process.

The task was intended to reinforce and affirm the women's sense of their own ability to cope, or self-efficacy. Witnessing and reflecting each other's problems and solutions in movement can deepen the empathy that is the foundation of mutual support. A variation on this task is outlined in Chapter 9 as a training exercise.

From the feedback women gave in program evaluations, one could infer that body image issues and the expression of emotion were salient. In the following examples people describe what they felt the benefits were:

> Learning that moving and breathing really does affect the body very much. We don't realize how much emotion we hold in.

> It's affirming, fun, relaxing, supportive, positive. No *invasive* body procedures!

> Taking time for myself – just to relax, move my body in a positive way – share things with the other group members. Getting in touch with my body – my new body – again.

The DMT interventions described in this section vary slightly in approach, methods, goals and settings. However, all attend to the emotional, psychological and social needs of women with breast cancer; all engage the mind/body connection in expressive movement processes; and all rely on the curative properties of group therapy. The empirical and anecdotal evidence gathered herein begs the question, why do women with breast cancer seem to respond so positively to DMT interventions? Possible explanations include the fact that most dance/movement therapists are women, and DMT methods may have evolved over time to affine well with the needs of female patients. As women, these breast cancer patients would tend to use support-oriented coping strategies anyway, and DMT groups clearly provide social support. Characteristics of the disease may contribute to DMT's impact. First, breast cancer strikes a clearly demarcated body site that is laden with personal, sexual and psychosocial meaning. Second, the initial surgical treatment, lumpectomy or mastectomy, alters the appearance of the breast and thus has immediate body image, social, sexual and/or relationship consequences. If we recall Vamos's (1993) identification of illness-related disruptions of appearance as a key component of body image difficulties, we may see perhaps that the need to address these issues may be stronger than with diseases for which the remedy is less disfiguring and visible. These possibilities are pure conjecture, but the clarification of any could inform the future practice of DMT with medical populations.

Dance/movement therapy in pediatric oncology

This review of DMT in the area of pediatric oncology includes the work published to date in the field, presented against a backdrop of theory and research in pediatric psychology. To begin, an understanding of how children experience and cope with cancer or other life-threatening childhood illnesses can inform the work of all therapists. As Kazak reported, "increased survival rates for childhood cancer have resulted in estimates that in 1990 1 of every 1,000 twenty-year-olds will be a survivor of childhood cancer" (Meadows and Silber 1985 as cited in Kazak 1989, para. 14). From this statistic one can infer that a similar proportion of adults in psychotherapy settings will have had cancer as children. The developmental perspective accepts that the experience will impact subsequent phases of life.

While cancer and its treatment can be seen as a trauma, recent advances in pediatric psychology and Child Life therapies have provided ways to ease the level of shock and distress associated with medical interventions and hospitalization. Rather, cancer can be seen as a "complex of stressors" to a child, from major disruptions in the normal developmental process to dealing with the life-threatening nature of the disease (Yuval 1997). Returning briefly to the social ecology model for understanding childhood illness (Kazak 1989), we are reminded of how crucial it is for the pediatric psychooncology therapist to take "both child and family into account in an additive, interactive and nonlinear sense. Within this model, the child's attributes, perceptions, understanding, and reactions interact with those of other family members" (Kazak 1989, para. 13). Kazak's view that "a systems perspective also incorporates processes over time" (para. 7) invites the DMT working in pediatric oncology to overlay the developmental framework on which our work relies with attention to school functioning, family, and social relationships. So far, pediatric medical DMT in hematology/oncology has focused exclusively on psychosocial and developmental adjustment, and not questions of any possible direct effects on disease processes.

The current state of the DMT specialty in pediatric medical work rests largely on the innovative work by the team at Tomorrow Children's Institute of Hackensack Medical Center (New Jersey), led by Susan Cohen, MA, CMA, ADTR, CCLS, Director of Creative Arts Therapies and Child Life Therapy in that hematology/oncology program. Cohen and Walco (1999) have articulated a developmental model of stress and adjustment that is grounded in social ecology theory and applied to DMT with child cancer patients. Beginning with infancy, Cohen has designed DMT assessment and intervention strategies that are developmentally sensitive, systems oriented and responsive to the cancer-related issues of her child patients. For example, Cohen's work in the PICU with a leukemic infant named Brad resembles Kasovac's PICU interventions (see Chapter 4) in the primary use of tactile stimulation. Cohen adds a focus on the auditory channel with music and vocal input, and props to form a developmentally appropriate visual and kinetic connection to an adult in dyadic interactions. Regarding the combined voice and touch approach, Cohen wrote:

> Through repetitive intervention of this nature, it was intended for Brad to experience his body boundaries, sense various connections between regions of his body by developing a sense of his own bodily organization, and experience containment in an environment that alternated between chaotic and restrictive extremes. (Cohen and Walco 1999, p.37).

This description brings to life developmental theory by Stern (1990) regarding the infant's need to develop receptive perceptual skills for relating to the environment, and Kestenberg (1975) regarding bodily organization as an initial task of infancy. Importantly, Cohen transferred the DMT activities to the baby's mother, who could begin to normalize the nascent relationship with her son through these modified modes of interaction.

Yuval (1997) discussed four foci for DMT with children who have cancer. They are presented here in terms of the cognitive, psychomotor and emotional aspects of the experience.

1. The creative modality makes the intangible, invisible aspect of cancer concrete and cognitively accessible with imaginary use of props and stories. This is especially important for children who have not yet attained Piaget's level of formal operations in cognitive development (see Bibance and Walsh 1980) (*cognitive* focus).

2. There is a feeling of betrayal by one's own body and body image is disturbed. Movement activities encourage a sense of mastery and control with the body (*psychomotor* focus).

3. In DMT, children express anger, fear and loss but also joy, happiness and hope. There is a joy in moving, and a feeling of wholeness (*emotional* focus).

4. In fantasy play and symbolism children can face threatening situations in non-threatening ways (*emotional* focus).

Adolescents, in particular, struggle with body image issues. According to Cohen and Walco (1999), "body image attitudes become negative, instilling even greater loss, passivity and withdrawal. Dance/movement therapy interventions that focus on mobilization, gross motor skills, and emotional self-expression aim to consolidate disease-related changes in the body and subsequent function" (Cohen and Walco 1999, p.40). Cohen's therapeutic support group for teens with cancer, "The Braves," designed their own game of indoor touch football, and this mobilized them in safe, age-appropriate ways. Teams were composed by gender, and the ongoing game became a "battle of the sexes" (Cohen and Walco 1999, p.40). In this way the teens could express their sexuality in a peer group of others who were experiencing the same challenges to autonomous functioning, self-concept and life itself.

Cancer can be fatal, and children with cancer become aware of the possibility of premature death in ways consistent with their level of cognitive and emotional development. Children's conceptions of death develop in the same stages as do their understanding of illness and hospitalizations. Fears of loneliness, separation and abandonment dominate the awareness of a child under the age of five. Children between six and ten years old know they are seriously ill and fear the loss of bodily integrity; and children ten and older have an overt awareness of and anxiety about impending death (La Greca and Stone 1985).

In DMT, children with cancer communicate their awareness and fears through symbolic activity. Mendelsohn's case description of an eight-year-old girl named Dana is an example (Mendelsohn 1999). Dana had a malignant brain tumor and was hospitalized for intensive chemotherapy treatments. In a DMT session with her grandfather present and observing, Dana playfully covered the therapist with scarves until she was invisible. Mendelsohn used her own subjective experience of suffocation while wrapped in the scarves to perceive and interpret the activity as a symbolic expression about death. She stayed in the imaginary mode with the child and responded to this verbally, saying "I can't breathe and can barely see. I'm scared... Where are you? Why are you leaving me here alone?..." (Mendelsohn 1999, p.76). In this intervention, the therapist tapped into the salient theme of aloneness: despite the presence of caring family members, the child was essentially alone in her illness and may have been anticipating the aloneness of death as well.

As Cohen and Walco noted, there is a need for systematic investigation of the benefits DMT may confer for children coping with cancer (1999). This author submits that the case reports and narratives easily justify continued use and exploration of DMT in pediatric oncology. These anecdotal data suggest that the modality provides a unique combination of therapeutic elements that are important for this population: developmental sensitivity, symbolism, play, creativity, mobilization and the centrality of the body orientation.

CHAPTER 6

Related Applications

This chapter is devoted to two related applications of dance/movement therapy (DMT) in the health care spectrum:

1.   work with families and caregivers

2.   work in the areas of death, dying and bereavement.

As with other psychosocial services in health care, the role of the dance/ movement therapist is not limited to the needs of patients themselves. From a systems perspective, we consider the needs of the family, loved ones and caregivers as well. This includes both personal caregivers, who are often family members, and professional caregivers. From a wholistic perspective, we assume our role in the system in the dimension of healing rather than curing, as outlined in Chapter 1. This is particularly important in the dying process, when cure is no longer a goal, but the focus is on comfort, separation and resolution.

Families and caregivers
Children of seriously ill parents
A study by Siegel, Karus and Raveis (1996) compared levels of depression and anxiety in children who were anticipating the death of a parent through cancer to a community sample of children who were not facing this stressor. They found that in the year preceding a parent's death from cancer, children show significantly higher levels of depression (as measured by Kovac's Children's Depression Inventory) and anxiety (measured by Speilberger's State–Trait Anxiety Scales for Children and Youth).

When a child learns that his or her parent has cancer, he or she begins to experience a host of reactions. Regardless of the prognosis, most of these children harbor a fear of losing the parent. In support groups they can learn they are not alone and express the myriad of emotions among other peers (Mancarella 2000). Wellness Community centers around the U.S. offer such groups in their Kids' Circle programs. The groups described in this chapter were co-led by this author with two clinical social workers, Michele Rossi and Minerva Lermond, and took place at the Wellness Community Delaware.

In this program, a ritualized session opening was developed. The leaders would begin by stating why the group meets: "Every child here has a parent who has or who has had cancer." Children then introduce themselves and tell basic information regarding the ill parent in whatever way they understand it: "My dad has cancer in his blood" or "My mom had breast cancer but now she is better" or "My mom died of cancer." Each child then takes a turn telling "one good thing and one bad thing" that has happened in the previous week. Their responses may or may not focus on the parent's illness, but allow the therapists to assess the children's need for containment, disclosure, or catharsis. Following this the therapists guide the children through structured tasks geared to expressing and communicating their feelings and needs. There is an emphasis on the curative group factors of universality and installation of hope (Yalom 1995). The vignettes are excerpted from the author's log, and illustrate how a blending of movement and verbal processes can contain the intensity of the children's feelings, and structure the need to communicate while channeling anxiety.

NAMING AND SHOWING THE FEELINGS

There were three girls and five boys in this group. One boy and two sisters had lost moms to cancer. Another mother (of a boy and a girl) had end-stage cancer and is in constant pain. The grandmother of two boys here had cancer metastasized to the kidney. Another mother had multiple brain tumors.

After the ritualized group opening, the children were given colorful index cards and asked to write down "one or just a few things you feel or think about the cancer or the person who has or had the cancer." They did not talk about these themes at that point. I simply collected them and kept them in my pocket during a movement warm-up. After the warm-up, the cards were returned to the children with instructions to get a partner and form each other into body sculptures to show one idea from the card. After the first "sculptors" made their statues, they titled them and showed them to the group. The children then switched roles. Themes were "Angry," "Sad," "Mad at God," "Praying". After everyone had made and shared the sculptures, there was a verbal discussion of feelings and thoughts, referring back to the movement task.

During a free play break at the end of the session one girl, Chelsea, asked to sculpt the adults. She shaped the social worker, and then me, into praying shapes. She positioned us facing each other closely and covered us with a blue scarf. She said the prayer was so we didn't hurt so much. I asked if we could pray that she doesn't hurt so much. She said yes. It was her mother with end-stage cancer.

ANGER AT THE CANCER

An eight-year-old boy, Michael, worked on this task with two therapists supporting his expression:

"If the cancer were an animal, what would it be?"

- A lion, because a lion eats other animals.
- A crab, because it can be painful.
- A snake, because it sneaks up on you...you never know when.

We drew the animal as a combination of the three: a big ugly "cancer monster". Then we pasted the picture on the wall.

"How do you feel when you see the lion-crab-snake cancer monster?"

Sad – scared – angry.

"What do you want to do in relation to it?"

- Run away.
- Punch it.
- Fight it.
- Throw things at it!
- Stop it!

We did all of those things, physically and vocally, directing punches and kicks and shouts to the picture – throwing foam balls. When Michael felt finished, he chose what to do with the cancer monster picture.

Wreck it...get rid of it.

And we did just that. The cancer monster was tossed out in the trash that day.

A CANCER DANCE/DRAMA

The group focused on information about cancer, and the social worker opened in a psycho-educational format, teaching basic facts about the white blood cells of the immune system, tumors and two types of treatment: radiation and chemotherapy. The children then enacted two versions of the cancer story in a dance/drama form, playing out the roles of cancer, the body, the patient and the treatments. The group included children who had lost a parent as well children with parents in treatment and parents in remission. It was important that everyone's experience be told in their dance, and not just the ones with the happy ending. Therefore, in the first version, the cancer won and the person died. In the second version, the cancer lost and the person was cured.

Large colored scarves served as simple costumes. Two children played the role of tumor or cancer cells and used dark colored scarves. (A child should not represent the cancer alone, for it is truly feared and hated in this population.) Two used light colored scarves to dance the part of the white blood cells. In green scarves, two represented the radiation treatment in an apt movement: bent forward at the waist as though skiing, with strong tension emanating towards the "patient" from the head and face, and arms bent at the elbows, fists vibrating. The child playing the chemotherapy ran about among the cancer cells and white blood cells. The "patient" called out when it was time for the next treatment, reacted to all treatments and the ebb and flow of the disease, and to the eventual outcome. When the make-believe death occurred, the feelings of sadness were authentic and given time for expression.

Later with his father present, Joey recalled how he was on the losing side in both versions of the dance/drama (first as the patient and then as the cancer). Together with his father, I told Joey that he can pretend losing in the Kids' Circle group activity and then in his real, everyday life he can win.

In this activity, the children took a process that is in reality out of their control and briefly took charge of it in a creative, interactive manner. Mastery is facilitated when children can embody and externalize stressful processes.

THE OBSTACLE COURSE OF CANCER

After the ritual opening, the social worker led a discussion to elicit and collect the children's questions about cancer. She clarified information misconceptions and planned to relay the children's thoughts to their parents. I then asked: "What do you have to go through – get through – deal with – when a parent has cancer?" and collected their answers: finding out, crying/feeling sad, feeling angry, being scared, worrying, doing more new chores at home, feeling alone.

Following a movement warm-up, we returned to these responses, and built a "cancer in the family obstacle course". Two kids made signs to label each "station", and four built the course using props. Joey choreographed "finding out" by crawling under a chair and through a hula hoop. For "feeling sad/crying," Jimmy sat in a chair wiping tears with a big blue cloth. To depict "worrying," Lisa paced in a circle around a chair biting her nails. Sarah showed "scared" by sitting in the middle of the space covered by a big cloth. For "feeling alone," one child crawled into the purple "bodysox" (a cocoon-like fabric prop in which a child can be completely surrounded, but still look out, and out of which he or she can easily crawl at will). The "feeling angry" part of the course was a place to make a lot of noise with a small collection of rhythm instruments. The station for "doing more chores" entailed picking up all the scarves and foam balls, then sweeping the floor in pantomime.

The signs were placed at each station, and the children all learned the movement patterns. Each child then moved through the course starting with finding out, but then using a sequence that he or she felt matched his or her own experience. "Everyone goes through it in their own way." When each child got to the end of the course, there was cheering, hugging and loud congratulations.

The children decided to keep the course up for their parents, and to show them how to go through. After the children showed their movements, the social worker invited any adults who wished to try. Joey and Chelsea, whose mother had died several months before, implored their dad to try, and he complied and went through. Spontaneously, Jimmy's dad, who had recurrent lymphoma, got up and went through the course. His wife and son and the other five families watched in silent support. The fathers, too, were loudly cheered and congratulated.

Parents of seriously ill children

The single session described below provides an example of how DMT might be a useful form of support to parents with seriously ill children. On invitation from the Department of Nursing, I led a one-time DMT-based support session at the Children's Hospital of Philadelphia for parents of children hospitalized on their inpatient units. The group was held during the coffee hour in their Connelly Family Research Center, so that the parents did not need to plan any extra time away from their children. The goals of the group were as follows:

- to offer dance/movement experience as a restorative resource for themselves

- to establish a group culture in order to encourage ongoing connection between the parents who participate and

- to educate parents about DMT as a resource.

The room filled with mothers and fathers, conversing over coffee and snacks. Some sat or stood alone. The mood varied from worried and withdrawn to social and bright. Some people seemed quite at home here, and some quite uncomfortable.

I announced that the group was starting and gave the verbal introduction loudly enough that everyone could hear and have the option of joining further. A few came closer. I put the music on, and over half of the people in the room participated in warm-ups that focused on tension release. When the session shifted to movement interaction and expression, four women gathered closer into the center area. I opened the expressive movement work by presenting these ideas:

1.   Parents are very good, expert even, at reading the nonverbal cues from their children. Even when the child can't talk, they can see and feel what they need: a drink, a hug, some space, etc.

2.   Perhaps with the child's illness you have become less attentive to you own bodily cues and your own felt needs.

3.   When parents take care of themselves, they can be more present for the children.

All four mothers nodded in agreement with these observations, then each introduced herself and shared some basic information about her sick child. The first movement task was to "think of your child and something that he or she needs. Embody that in a movement. Explore it and repeat until it feels like a representation of what they feel and need." For the most part, the women explored this movement theme with eyes closed. When each had "found" her movement phrase, we took the group focus around the circle and joined each mother by doing the phrase with her, affirming her expression by reflecting it back. One mother of an infant girl made swaying, rocking movements. Another lifted her arms as in worship or prayer. The mother of a ten-year-old boy threw an imaginary baseball, caught it, and threw it, again and again. She cried quietly while she did this and while she showed it to the group. I offered the suggestion that we are all throwing and playing a little baseball for him now, until he can get out there and play on his own again.

The second task asked the moms to tune in to themselves, to breathe deeply and "pay attention to what you feel you need right now, these days, in this time. It can be very concrete or very abstract. Embody that in a movement or movements that express and represent what *you* need." The mother of the baby girl closed her eyes, hugged herself and swayed in place. One woman began the movement of taking a shower. She took a whole imaginary shower using lots of self-touch and the indulging Effort qualities of *lightness* and *sustainment*. Again, these movements and the ideas in them were shared all around, repeated and reflected with the woman who created it.

The final task was to "try combining the two. Go back and forth between the movements about what the child needs and the movements about what you need, until you find a way for them to fit together…a way of knowing that you can both get your needs met…that there is a way to do this. Play with how they flow from one to the other…how the movements are connected and how you and your child are connected right now."

When the women emerged from this private exploration of the two movement phrases, I led the group to closure standing and coming together in a circle. The women initiated holding hands. I suggested that we close in such a way that people can affirm the work they've done today and be available for each other in the future. Someone in the group suggested praying and I gently redirected this to structure a moment of silence in which each can "say in her heart and mind what she wishes and needs to say." During this there were tears and very tender verbal expressions. I acknowledged their obvious strength as they had maintained a generous attention to each other and the feelings that morning, wished them continued strength and their children health. Their need for support and self-care that morning must have been great, for these four women participated in this dance/movement group in a setting with many distractions.

Siblings of ill children

Systems theory would predict that when a child is seriously ill, the other children in the family will be impacted. It follows that these children would benefit from psychosocial support that is developmentally sensitive. Lotan-Mesika (2000) reviewed the literature on the psychosocial needs of siblings of seriously ill children. It may be summarized as follows: siblings experience disequilibrium and many new stressors as they participate in new activities and try to find their place in a shifting and challenged system. Their own fears and sadness are connected to the facts that they will live the longest with the memories of the illness, however it may conclude, and that they may identify with their sibling. They may feel unnoticed by and isolated from their parents who are concentrating their energies on the needs of the sick child. They have been asked to be kind and considerate of their ill brother or sister yet they may feel jealous, and confused by their own feelings. Lotan-Mesika cites a call for programming that will provide emotional, informational, instrumental and self-appraisal support to these children (Murray 1999, in Lotan-Mesika 2000, p.16).

Along with Toni Freni, ADTR, Lotan-Mesika co-led a series of DMT sessions for child siblings of pediatric oncology patients at the Tomorrow's Children's Institute. The responses of a 12-year-old boy named Josh exemplify the potential of the modality for providing the necessary support. This sequence took place in his second session, during an activity with the stretch-band, a large circular loop of stretchy, flexible fabric:

> While the group was exploring the stretch-band, Josh wanted to take the responsibility of "holding" all group members as they were leaning on it. The therapist inquired about Josh's general perception of his responsibilities. Josh said that he does a lot of things at home, for example: clean the bathroom, wash the dishes. Josh's movements appeared disparate from the group's synchrony and common rhythm, as he was pulling, pushing and moving against the direction of the other group members' movements. However, when he had the opportunity to be in the center of the circle he seemed more contained and calm, as well as bound and restricted. (Lotan-Mesika 2000, p.110)

It appears that Josh had a need to communicate about his experience. In the movement, he displayed contrasting themes (wanting to hold the group, then clashing with the group, then calming and restraining himself when the focus of the group), perhaps as a manifestation of his ambivalence, or his own conflicting wants and needs during his brother's illness.

Multifamily formats

Multifamily groups are not uncommon in mental health settings. This format recognizes the primacy of the family system while building a sense of community around a shared challenge. For families dealing with serious illness, this is especially important as it combats the family's sense of isolation and gives an opportunity for the exchange of information, coping strategies and support. In multifamily work using the creative arts therapies, children can contribute equally and competently with their parents. This is in contrast to strictly verbal sessions, where their less developed language skills may put them at a disadvantage compared to the adults. Two examples of collaborations between social work and DMT follow to illustrate how movement experiences provide a vehicle for safe communication about feelings and conflicts.

DMT Pat Mowry Rutter and her social work colleague ran a multifamily group for the families of children with severe asthma at National Jewish Medical Center (Mowry Rutter, personal communication, July 18, 2002). The group, composed of four families at a time, would include the patients, their parents and their siblings. The social worker would open the group with a discussion of the illness, then Mowry Rutter would direct an adapted movement choir, a communally oriented group improvisational movement form developed by Laban (Bartenieff 1980, p.139). This structure, says Mowry Rutter, works quickly to get to the important issues in a family. The movers would be asked, "How do you feel right now?" Each person then made a single, simple movement phrase based on that feeling. Everyone would learn all the movements created in the group and this would start laughter or elicit strong emotions. Soon someone would be able to describe the movement or the feeling in a word. Often this was emotional language, revealing angers or frustrations that people had been denying even to themselves. A parent might disclose, "This kid is ruining my life. I have to have a 15-year-old sleeping in my room in case they stop breathing."

As Lotan-Mesika (2000) also discussed, sometimes siblings of the asthmatic children can feel jealous and hurt because the sick child's needs dominate the focus of the family, and the family's development is disrupted (Mowry Rutter, July 18, 2002). Brothers and sisters may be required to live under the same behavioral restrictions as those the asthmatic child needs, and they may respond with rebellious acting out. The multifamily groups became a venue for appropriate communication of these frustrations and dynamics.

Occasional multifamily groups in the Wellness Community's Kids' Circle program gave the parents a chance to join their children in creative expressive activity. This is how one such session with four families transpired.

The social worker led a drawing task wherein each family created a sociogram showing how the family is embedded in an interacting network of people and support, and then embellished it with images and symbols of each person or element. The task is reminiscent of Kazak's (1989) social-ecological theoretical framework. After each family shared their drawing with the group, I extended the theme into movement, with a focus on appreciation and coping.

"Notice all the people in the drawing. Notice how the people who are here with you today are pictured there. Think about the people with you here today and think of one thing about them that you love…one thing about that person that helps you get through the tough times." From there I structured a statue-making task, asking each family to make a sculpture of each person, showing that characteristic. As a model, I sculpted my colleague into a big "belly laugh" statue to represent her sense of humor.

Timmy's father sculpted him into a posture lying on the floor drawing. "When you're feeling low, Timmy will draw a picture and bring it to you, and it helps me feel better."

The parents of a resilient teenage girl sculpted her into a position that mimed sitting on the phone talking. They spoke about how she went on growing and living and being a normal girl, and this helped them both through the mother's breast cancer treatment.

Brian, whose father had died only three weeks before, took a long time moving his mother about, and with some guidance shaped a "hugging/talking" sculpture. He put himself in it – a two-person sculpture with the two of them sitting and facing each other, arms on the other's shoulders, foreheads nearly touching, eye to eye. There was no interpretation needed. He saw his mother as close and connected to him.

In these sculptures, children and parents found nonverbal ways of expressing support and caring for each other. The task also reinforced positive aspects of the families' coping style.

Professional caregivers

One pilot study (Russell 1996) examined the potential of DMT to remediate occupational stress among health care workers, specifically female nurses working in long-term pediatric inpatient care units. Using the psychometrically sound Strain Questionnaire (SQ) by Lefebvre and Sandford (1985, as cited in Russell 1996) she measured self-reported stress in a pre-test–post-test design. DMT-based stress reduction sessions included a body-oriented warm-up, stretching, relaxation with guided imagery, improvisational creative movement processes, and verbal exchanges about the movement experiences. Using a Mann-Whitney U test, this author compared pre-test to post-test change scores in Russell's experimental and control groups. Total SQ change was significantly greater in the intervention group than in the control group (U= 1, p=.043), with the intervention group showing more reduction of self-reported stress. The sample size was small (N=8) and the findings tentative, but should encourage more research on the value of DMT for the well-being of health care providers who experience occupational stress.

Death, dying and bereavement

Patients who are dying

Terminally ill patients need care that is oriented to healing rather than curing. This is known as palliative care, which is an umbrella concept for services that aim to reduce discomfort and pain and to help people address psychological, relational and spiritual issues as they prepare for a dignified and peaceful death. Hospice care is part of the palliative care spectrum, and may occur in hospitals or nursing homes, in patients' homes or in special hospice facilities. The medical priority is for pain control, which may include the use of medications, radiation treatments or blood transfusions. Palliative care is concerned with quality of life, and acknowledges the end of life as an essential phase for health care attention. It is worth noting that spiritual well-being may provide a protective buffer against the depression that can erode quality of life for the terminally ill (Nelson et al. 2002), when spirituality is understood as an individual's intrinsic seeking of meaning in life, illness or death. There is an untested premise in palliative care that one should stay open to the terminally ill patient's or family member's own inclinations to include spiritual elements in the process, and remain supportive yet neutral regarding specific religious affiliations or practices (Nelson et al. 2002). The DMT case examples and perspectives included in this chapter manifest that premise.

DMT skills and methods enrich hospice care therapy in the establishment of relationships, assessment of needs, and strengthening of the patient's positive resources. Since 1989, Linni Deihl, ADTR, has expanded her extensive work in DMT to hospice care for people dying of cancer, AIDS, or other illnesses (personal communication, July 22, 2002). In an interview conducted for the purposes of this text, she explained the nature of hospice care and how it dovetails with DMT. Hospice services through Long Island's East End Hope for Hospice agency, where

Deihl is employed as a dance/movement therapist, begin when a patient's life expectancy is assessed at six months or less. Services continue until after the death, when Deihl continues to counsel the family through the initial bereavement period. In the months and weeks leading up to the death, the hospice therapist helps demystify the dying process for family members, and supports them as they cope with multiple stressors. Deihl describes her hospice work as structurally quite different from conventional DMT and psychotherapeutic work: she sees one patient at a time in the patient's home, four hours per week, until the patient's death.

These are long therapeutic relationships that begin, as expected, with the establishment of safety and trust. Deihl's focus here is to learn what the patient most needs, whether physical, practical, emotional or relational. She is joining the patient "on the last leg of their life's journey" and this begins with an identification of "life's gifts," to strengthen the patient's sense of the positive aspects of life remembered and life remaining (Deihl, personal communication, July 22, 2002). The psychological focus may then shift to "uncover" the negative or unfinished issues. Deihl sees the therapist's role here not as a catalyst for behavioral change but, for instance, to help the patient examine a problematic relationship and to help the patient prepare for the dialogues with his or her loved ones that will "mend fences." The goal is to permit a death that is unfettered by conflict, guilt or unexpressed feelings. Helping someone prepare to die may entail the use of other psychotherapeutic structures. Deihl describes how one woman expressed her overwhelming anxiety and anger through constant, unproductive talking, reviewing her life and feelings so relentlessly that people in her life were turned away. To channel her feelings and help her organize the chaotic expression, Deihl helped the patient make an audio-journal, a record for her family. Later, her cassette tapes were transcribed and made into a book with pictures for her family.

Deihl's work with terminally ill patients is highly reliant on movement observation and assessment. Hospice patients may be bedridden or confined to a chair, and there may be little gross motor movement. This requires sensitivity to subtle initiations and qualitative changes. Incongruent verbal and nonverbal expressions signal to Deihl that there may be an unresolved issue associated with the topic. This will be explored and will provide a point of entry to the psychological work described above. When patients become unable to speak, the nonverbal channel becomes the only available form of interaction. Consistent with all movement therapy, the relationship is formed in movement and Deihl describes using the standard DMT techniques of reflecting posture, gesture and/or movement dynamics continually throughout her lengthy sessions. The therapist's attunement to the patient's mind/body state, or "body empathy," may mitigate the sense of isolation and fear experienced by the dying, and humanizes the dying process (Deihl 1992). These competencies, movement assessment and body empathy, are discipline-specific to DMT, and represent a unique contribution of the specialty to hospice care.

There are distinct warm-up, theme development and closure segments in Deihl's hospice sessions, albeit stretched over a very long time frame and less formally structured than in psychotherapy sessions. Perhaps it is the profoundly intimate quality of body empathy that enables Deihl to describe how despite the intensity of the work with dying patients, there is a sense of more time and freedom to let the therapeutic relationship develop slowly. In this author's view, there is an intriguing paradox: in one reality hospice patients actually have very little time left, and yet, in the therapy, there is a sense of there being a lot of time. This feature of the hospice work, body empathy, may constitute one of its healing factors.

Deihl sees the hospice work as a way to honor life. She tells her hospice patients, "What an honor it was to be present at this point in their lives, and what a gift they were to me, and how much they were going to give to me as well as what I would give to them" (Deihl, personal communication, July 22, 2002).

Cohen (1996) also identifies "kinesthetic empathy" as central to the DMT of terminally ill children. Two developmental factors make the already tragic nature of a child's death even more difficult. When well, children live more mobile and physically active lives than do adults. They rely on their bodies for catharsis and self-expression. When the body begins to fail, the ability to release tension and express themselves is seriously compromised. Second, psychological development towards an autonomous identity is in progress (Kestenberg 1975) and the child's attachment to loving adults is central to mental and physical health. Cohen explains the dance/movement therapist's particular resources for supporting a child through the dying process:

> As the therapist observes and describes the non-verbal cues, the child gains a better grasp of his or her feelings. Dying means separating and, ultimately, departure-transition from the familiar and comfortable to the unknown. By helping to open communication and self-examination in an important non-verbal way, the dance/movement therapist helps the child reach closure and confront the loneliness of having to say a final good-bye. (Cohen 1996, p.5)

Mind/body work may help people prepare for death by reducing some of the anxiety. In the project with cystic fibrosis adults described in Chapter 4 (Goodill 1995) one usually highly strung and anxious man emerged from deep relaxation and said, "Well, if my death is anything like that, maybe it won't be so bad."

Dancer/choreographer Bill T. Jones (1998), clear that his work is art and not therapy, nonetheless describes poignant and no doubt therapeutic sequences from his Survival Workshops (subtitled "Moving and Talking about Death") (Jones 1998, p.9). In these workshops, terminally ill teens and adults expressed their thoughts and feelings about their illness and impending deaths using imagery, words, structured dance/movement tasks and artwork. As planned, the workshops resulted in Jones's full-length dance theatre piece, "Still/Here," but he observed the inherently life-enhancing benefits of creative processes and group experience:

> Something else happened as well, people became more complicated and clear. They were breaking apart and rearranging themselves. They were sharing with each other, coining terms, making declarations, giving and receiving advice. At least two fell in love and are now married. I am convinced this richness was fueled by movement. (Jones 1998, p.11)

Melsom (1999) used DMT techniques to assist in the dying process with a 39-year-old woman, Sophia, who had suffered a stroke after surgery for a brain tumor. In the last few days of her life, she was left without speech and with voluntary movement only in her eyes, her head and one forearm. The session Melsom described included Sophia, and her twin sister, who was almost always at her side. The following is a direct quote from Melsom's report:

> Sophia and her sister held hands, and the sister was always keeping eye contact with Sophia. I commented on their non-verbal communication and how they seemed to have such a strong bond. I suggested that the sister take part in the session, and she responded very positively. I guided the two sisters in a non-verbal hand-dance, where they were taking turns: first one leading in the movement and the other following, and then switching roles. As they were engaged in this highly communicative hand-dance, the two sisters exchanged innumerable "silent" messages of compassion and love through their eyes. The sister complimented Sophia on her strength in the situation, and I encouraged the non-verbal expression of the strength though suggesting that they could hold each other's hands firmly. This use of physical strength, in the only body part she could move voluntarily, was facilitated in order to enhance a sense of control in an otherwise physically helpless situation. Sophia started to cry, and I verbally acknowledged how hard this situation must be for her. The sister said that Sophia had been afraid to cry because of swellings in the brain, caused by the tumor... This emotional release from Sophia elicited crying in her sister as well. Following was a period where the two sisters cried. No words were exchanged, only [this] sharing, in the presence of a witness, the dance/movement therapist. After a

while, we talked about the value of touch, and I suggested for the sister to gently massage Sophia's hands, or other body parts that were comfortable for her, as an interaction for the two of them during the day... As the sister was commenting on the fact that she was "holding her breath", I asked them both to focus on their breathing. I asked if they could breathe together, and modeled this. Gradually, they ended up sharing the same rhythm, and all three of us were breathing in synchrony. The calm atmosphere proceeded naturally to a closure. I asked if we could make a hand gesture saying good-bye to one another. Their hand gestures clearly carried emotions expressing their awareness that the final good-bye was imminent. (Melsom 1999, pp.183–4, reprinted with permission)

Bereavement

After the death of his wife, the English writer C. S. Lewis described the physicality of grief. He writes, "No one ever told me that grief felt so much like fear. I am not afraid, but the sensation is like being afraid. The same fluttering in the stomach, the same restlessness, the yawning. I keep on swallowing" (Lewis 1961, p.1). And later, "There is one place where her absence comes locally home to me, and it is a place I can't avoid. I mean my own body" (Lewis 1961, p.12). Lewis's poignant words show how the mind/body connection is very much a part of the grief experience.

The loss of a spouse or intimate partner may, in fact, pose a health risk for the surviving bereaved person. Research has found an association between bereavement and loss and diminished immune system functioning, with natural killer (NK) cell activity and cellular immunity (the work of the T-cells and macrophages) most affected (Berkman 1995; Kemeny 1994; Parham 2000; Schneiderman and Baum 1991). This effect should not be surprising if, as Lewis's description suggests, grief is like fear. When prolonged, the fear-like grief state would resemble chronic stress at the physiological level, and would lead to the same kinds of health threats discussed earlier in relation to stress. Accordingly, it becomes the responsibility of health care and human service providers to care for the loved ones of a dying or recently deceased patient. Bereavement services should be seen on a continuum of care following support groups like those described above. Fitzgerald (2000) has reported such work in a blended DMT and psycho-educational program for adults with developmental disabilities who are grieving.

The bereavement process unfolds in ways that are individual, but also sequential. Murphy (1985) synthesized a number of prevailing theories regarding the stages of grief (including the familiar framework by Elizabeth Kübler Ross)

(Kübler Ross 1969), to propose a wholistic model. It progresses from an initial *muted awareness* (feelings of numbness and shock) to a *defensive stage* (where there may be a clinging to the lost one or conversely, a dismissal of the importance of the loss). From there, Murphy describes a stage of *profound sadness* that resembles depression but is normal and necessary, not pathological. "The outcome of this stage is the maximally tolerable knowledge of the implications of and the extent of the loss..." (Murphy 1985, p.12). In Murphy's *recovery stage*, there is an acceptance of the loss and a recovery. In what she calls the *growth stage* there is a return to hope and affirmation of life, and in a final *transcendence stage* (achieved by some), there is a sense of connection to the universe and an opening up to new experience.

Murphy maintains that in grieving there are opportunities for rediscovering the self, and deepening one's capacities for intimacy.

> Pain, uncertainty, loneliness and helplessness are conditions of life. But grief also allows us to go beyond pain, helplessness and loneliness to creative resynthesis of ideas, to new emotional depth, and to a quickened appreciation of life and its connectedness. (Murphy 1985, p.14)

The DMT-based bereavement work developed by Judith Bunney, ADTR, manifests Murphy's thesis. In workshops entitled Honoring Life's Passages™ (J. Bunney, personal communication, July 15, 2002) Bunney addresses bereavement issues at the body level. Participants are asked to recall the loss at a physical level, to find postures and movement phrases that recreate and represent the experience of the loss (Bunney 2000). Bunney then gently guides the mover to move on and away from the loss. Using the simple movement structure, "Looking back and Moving forward" (© J. Bunney 2001), Bunney provides an elegant movement metaphor for the bereavement process. Participants travel on a diagonal pathway through space, or on curving pathways, for these have a soft and indulgent property. Bunney will often walk with the movers' slow strides, moving with them at their pace, but off to the side and not in direct reflection of the movement (see Sandel 1993b). People find this non-intrusive and supportive. They look back and acknowledge the lost one, and then turn to travel on, and as this pattern repeats the activity becomes an individual embodiment of the bereavement process.

Participants in the workshops are often self-referred mental health professionals and bereavement counselors themselves who come knowing that their own issues of grief and loss need to be deeply addressed in order for them to do their work in a healthy way. They may be novice or experienced movers. Bunney observes that novice movers can favor positions rather than movement, but it is the active, felt movement that is critical to the working through of loss. If someone "gets stuck" in a position and feels unable to move, Bunney will gently suggest that the position be experienced with more intensity or exaggeration so that part of the process can be transformed and then moving forward can begin. There also can be anger in the grieving process, and in the movement workshops, jumping or running with movement qualities of strength and quickness (what Laban called the *fighting elements*) might express the anger.

C. S. Lewis located the grief in his own body: "...where her absence comes locally home to me," he said (Lewis 1961, p.12). Bunney has observed that for people who have lost spouses or intimate partners, the loss of shared touch is the central theme. Sometimes in the workshops, people express the need to be held, missing the touch and the physical presence of the person who has died. This was true also for a participant whose husband was paralyzed. Even though he was still alive and could talk with her, she grieved the loss of his touch, and the quality of her touching him, where there now was a deadness in his inability to respond to her.

The workshops also emphasize ritual, as an element of spirituality and as a psychological container for the intensity of emotions and vulnerability that can accompany the movement experience. In this way, Bunney's work is a microcosm of the grieving process. For opening and closure, she uses the circle formation, which is also a container, and she recommends the use of musical accompaniment to support the strong emotions that will surface. Spiritual awareness must be part of the work, Bunney advises, and the lighting of candles is a nearly universal ritual to invite that awareness, but without attachment to any particular religious tradition.

Bereaved children

The aforementioned study by Siegel, Karus and Raveis (1996) conducted follow-up assessments of bereaved children 7 to 12 months after the death of a parent from cancer, and discovered a resilient pattern of response. These children, after an undeniably distressing experience and a profound loss, showed normal levels of anxiety and depression. The researchers cite other findings (Weller *et al.* 1999 cited in Siegel *et al.* 1996) that in the three- to twelve-week period following the death of a parent, children aged between five and twelve years met diagnostic criteria for a major depressive episode. Thus, it seems that the psychological well-being of bereaved children is most vulnerable in the first few months following the death. The 1996 study by Siegel and colleagues used measures of general psychological functioning, not grief-specific assessments, and the researchers allow that important issues may have thus been overlooked. They concluded, "the value of supportive therapy should not be overlooked because of the apparent resilience of children" (Siegel *et al.* 1996, para. 32).

Given that bereaved children do experience distress in the first months after losing a parent, the Wellness Community program permits children to continue in its Kids' Circle groups even after a parental loss due to cancer. The child and parent can decide together how long to keep attending groups. As one father said, to keep coming gives the bereaved children a sense of continuity in their lives. The following vignettes illustrate the usefulness of continuing involvement in support groups, and how DMT interventions can be integrated in multidisciplinary programming for these children.

GIVING AND TAKING SUPPORT

Chelsea and Joey's mom had just died. Their dad brought them to the Kids' Circle group one week after the death and three days after the funeral. Clearly this is their support. So, five of the eight children in the group today (Chelsea, Joey, Brad and his little brother Timmy, and Anna) have lost their mothers. Right at the beginning, Chelsea and Joey told the group about their mother's death. Most of the children were lying tummy-down during the brief verbal opening section of group. The movement warm-up started right from this position, with slow stretches to come halfway up from the floor. The children needed the support of the floor, and they needed to feel support from each other as well.

I structured a partner stretch: sitting back to back and taking turns slowly leaning forward to support the partner's back stretch. Kids paired up with their siblings for the most part. I worked directly with Chelsea and Joey, who were testy and complaining with each other in the beginning. With verbal encouragement and hands-on guidance they finally relaxed into supporting one another. The adults knew how in the years to come this brother and sister would need to sense and support each other in many ways. We gave them much praise for being able to quietly and sensitively do that today at the physical level.

LEARNING TO REMEMBER

As it turned out, all of the kids who came today, Brad and Timmy, Joey and Chelsea, have lost moms and the group leaders decided on a theme of grief for the group meeting. It was an organically evolving session that shifted from primarily verbal to primarily movement foci. Using a flip chart, the social worker elicited and recorded the children's descriptions of grief. Expressions included: sad, angry, relieved, wanting to hold onto memories. Brad said, "Everything feels blank in the world," and later, "Everything about them that you still have is precious and you should hold onto it."

Each child was asked to share a memory of his or her mother. Joey told about how their mom made up a "hide and then chase me" type game they used to play around the house. Then, the group actually played Joey's mom's game. Joey and his sister coached us all as we ran, squealed, dodged each other, and learned the funny toe-tagging that was part of it. Afterwards the group sat quietly, thought of their mother using her full name, and thanked her in our minds for a great game and a great memory. The children brought their mother's game back to life, made a good memory alive and made it their own.

To wrap up, each child drew a picture of a memory, and they invested in this task with quiet intensity. They brought their pictures to a circle around a lit candle and each told about his or her drawing. Sitting around the candle, arms around each other's shoulders, the group took two big breaths and then a third to blow the candle out together. The children suggested that the group always end this way.

Bunney (personal communication, July 15 2002) recommends that all dance/ movement therapists would benefit from exploring issues of grief and loss at the movement level. It is not easy, Bunney advises, because it is connected to one's own death. There is a natural fear and resistance to the notion of our own mortality. Yet, inasmuch as most of our mental health clients find themselves working through losses of various sorts during the therapeutic process, this will allow dance/movement therapists to support them in a clearer and more authentic way. In our professional lives as therapists, we also occasionally experience the death of our patients, possibly even by suicide. In the medical arena issues of threatened, impending or actual loss are almost always in one's consciousness. When dealing with the unknown – waiting for a diagnostic test or a prognosis, waiting for the end of a surgery, struggling with choices in the treatment plan – patients can experience fear and panic. It is about the possibility of death, and the therapist needs to be prepared to help.

In any health care field, clinical work is supported by theory, research and education (Chaiklin 1994). The creative and valuable DMT applications described in Part II are the products of many resourceful and inspired therapists who have extended their DMT training into the medical sphere. For most, this has been a nearly autonomous process of discovery, advocacy and independent learning. For the field to advance confidently as a specialty option for medical psychosocial services, educational programming and research priorities need to be articulated and pursued. In Part III, suggestions and proposals for this development are given.

Part III

Research and Education

CHAPTER 7

Research Issues in Medical Dance/Movement Therapy

Art and science are two sides of the same coin.
Art is a passion pursued with discipline
science is a discipline pursued with passion.

Arthur M. Sackler (1984), physician, psychobiology researcher
and arts philanthropist

This chapter considers a research agenda for medical dance/movement therapy (DMT) by presenting several potential research questions and topics, followed by a discussion of methodological issues for medical DMT. Selected studies from the current body of knowledge will be included. The chapter is not an introduction to DMT research, and assumes the reader's familiarity with basic clinical research principles. For a good overview of research options in the DMT literature, see Berrol (2000). At this time the body of work is nascent, with a handful of published and/or graduate-level projects. The existing work will thus be framed as examples and as the foundation for research efforts in the future.

For the reader who is familiar with recent discussions regarding the appropriateness of experimental research in the creative arts therapies (see Higgens 2001), it will soon be clear that most of the recommendations herein do lean towards the quantitative end of the spectrum. This emphasis is not to suggest in any way that human science approaches, such as phenomenological, heuristic, artistic, or ethnographic inquiry, do not hold value for medical DMT (see Creswell 1998; Giorgi 1985; Wadsworth Hervey 2000). On the contrary, these methods could address important questions regarding the process and techniques of therapy in medical settings, and some of the professional issues, from the therapists' perspectives. The field of nursing in particular has made impressive developments in qualitative research for health care questions. My objective in the present discussion is to highlight ways that medical DMT researchers can respond to requirements for evidence-based information about the modality's benefits for medical patients. This requirement is linked to larger issues such as patient access to services, third-party coverage of services, and positioning of the field for the acquisition of research funding on a par with other psychosocial specialties in health care.

Methods such as meta-analysis will be appropriate for that undertaking. Cruz and Sabers (1998) conducted a meta-analysis of aggregated effect size in a group of 16 studies of DMT with a range of populations and outcome variables. Their findings indicated a success rate of approximately 30 per cent for people treated with DMT over untreated individuals, an effect size that is comparable to that for other psychosocial therapies. As of this writing, there are too few studies of medical DMT applications to warrant meta-analysis and it would be premature to propose this kind of work at this time. Ultimately though, as the specialty develops and more studies are published, it will be important to aggregate the findings in order to make overall conclusions about the effectiveness of DMT with medical patients.

Achterberg included a dance metaphor in this broad-based yet practical appreciation of research and science:

> Science, when well practiced, is a ballet of discovery, an elegant accoutrement to the rest of the world's knowledge. More important, it provides a prohibition on self-delusion, which distinguishes the scientific methods of observation from other ways of seeking information. (Achterberg 1985, p.8)

Proposed medical dance/movement therapy research priorities

Throughout this volume, various foci for medical DMT research have been suggested. These span questions to inform assessment, treatment and outcome issues. They are compiled and presented below, with a few additions.

Assessment in medical DMT

According to Green (1985) psychosocial assessment of medical patients is both more abbreviated and more extensive than standard mental health assessment. The assessment focuses on the relationships between psychosocial factors and the current medical condition. The goal of the medical psychosocial assessment is to move from "the construction of a clinical syndrome" (Green 1985, p.134) towards the "development of a preventive or remedial plan" (Green 1985, p.133). The clinician needs to appraise recent events, environmental and relational resources, and premorbid personality factors in the context of the medical circumstances. This necessitates a systems approach to the task: "Clinical analyses must not only systematically evaluate these varied elements but must also elucidate their interrelationships and dynamic flow" (Green 1985, p.133). The data for such an assessment is gathered from overt behaviors and the patient's own expression of feelings, the family's expression of feelings and stressors, and known biophysical processes that may be influencing mental status. The clinician inquires about the patient's current stressors, and about attitudes towards both the illness and the health care he or she is receiving. Questions regarding spirituality should be part of the assessment. From this the clinician attempts to elucidate any developmental influences on the current problems and makes inferences regarding intrapsychic processes that may play a role in the disease or recovery processes (Green 1985).

Green cautioned that psychosocial assessment should not burden the medically ill patient, whose mental and physical resources are strained. "Brevity, clarity and minimal intrusiveness maximize patient compliance and minimize fatigue" (Green 1985, p.135). DMT assessment makes maximum use of the individual's spontaneous nonverbal behaviors as an information-gathering method, and thus meets Green's criteria of minimal intrusiveness and low patient burden. Throughout this volume, clinical anecdotes have illustrated the dance/movement therapist's use of movement observation skills in the process of treatment planning.

Unlike our colleagues in health psychology and medical social work, medical dance/movement therapists do not have assessment instruments that are validated specifically for specialty use with medical populations. One such instrument, however, is under development and worth mentioning as a model for future clinical assessment research in DMT. Serlin's Kinaesthetic Imaging Profile (SKIP) is designed for use with women with breast cancer. Serlin and colleagues (2000; Serlin 1999b) began with a qualitative, inductive approach using in-depth interviews with the women in their program, and drew on the language the women used to describe their bodily felt experiences with cancer and in the DMT program. From this pool of descriptors, Serlin has developed a self-report checklist that is currently being tested for validity and reliability. The second arm of the SKIP is a movement observation component based in Laban Movement Analysis (LMA), and derived from observations by Serlin and other trained movement specialists over several groups of women in her DMT program. The combination of movement assessment and self-report elements should yield an instrument that is specific and sensitive to the mind/body aspects of the breast cancer experience. The authors intend that the tool will be sensitive to therapeutic change brought about by DMT and serve as an outcome measure for future research. The depth, specificity and rigor invested in the development of Serlin's instrument are comparable to the processes of instrument development in the larger field of health psychology, making the SKIP a landmark in the establishment of medical DMT as a specialty.

There are other outstanding questions about psychological assessment through movement in the context of medical illness. Diagnostic research and clinical observation using LMA have noted that in states of unhealth, such as depression (Davis 1991) and in debilitated conditions due to primary medical illness (Diehl 1992), the Efforts go "neutral". They seem to diminish or disappear from the movement repertoire. Flow Effort is the substrate for the other Effort elements and Amighi *et al.* (1999) describe neutral flow as appearing "inanimate, either limp like a rag doll or stiff like a robot... This is because Neutral Flow reflects an absence of vitality and a numbing of emotions and thoughts" (Amighi *et al.* 1999, p.25). Indeed, the experience of moving without effort, without the *antrieb* or "inner impulse to move" (Bartenieff 1980), is mechanical and flat. To inform medical DMT assessment methods, this question could be researched in observational studies using correlational and/or longitudinal designs. For example, a longitudinal design might best involve patient participants with chronic disease conditions that have episodic patterns. Examples might be cystic fibrosis, or autoimmune problems like systemic lupus erythematosus (or SLE, also commonly called "lupus"). Observations conducted during periods of relatively better health could be compared to observations during flare-ups of the disease. This way, personality variables can be differentiated from whatever movement features may appear during periods of acute illness.

Self-efficacy

The reader will recall that self-efficacy, the belief in one's capacity to act on one's own behalf, can be bolstered through interactive and social interventions that encourage independent activity. DMT may be particularly effective for increasing self-efficacy. In DMT the patient is active, and the therapy proceeds based on the patient's initiations. These features set the modality apart from other mind/body methods where the patient may be still (as in sitting meditation and relaxation), passive to the practitioner's ministrations (as in massage therapy or therapeutic touch), or led through set movement sequences (as in yoga, tai chi or Qi-gong). Bartenieff emphasized the connection between the patient's intent to act and his or her "independent participation" in recovery through movement (Bartenieff

1980, p.3). DMT outcome studies focusing specifically on self-efficacy as a dependent variable are recommended to explore this notion. An example of such research is Brauninger's (2000) ongoing study of DMT for stress management and quality of life in which "self-effectiveness" is one outcome variable.

Quality of Life

As outlined in Chapter 1, health related quality of life (HRQOL) is relevant in acute and chronic conditions and in terminal illness; for patients, family members and caregivers; and across the lifespan. For DMT and other psychosocial services in health care, quality of life is an overall objective of our work. In a National Institutes of Health report on complementary and alternative therapies, quality of life is identified as especially important for clinical and research focus (Cassileth, Jonas and Cassidy 1994). Dibbel-Hope (2000) and Serlin *et al.* (2000) gathered data about various aspects of HRQOL in their studies of DMT for women with breast cancer. Brauninger's (2000) project is another example of DMT research with this focus, although not necessarily with medically ill study participants. Dozens of quality of life measurement instruments have been developed and validated, and are specific to many health care conditions. It is recommended that medical DMT clinical outcome studies include quality of life as an outcome variable and, if possible, utilize a measurement tool that is validated for the population under study. This way, the effectiveness of DMT in the general health arena can be compared to other modalities.

Adherence

Adherence to self-care regimens is critical to health for adults, teens and children with all types of chronic conditions and for those in medical rehabilitation. The literature presented in this volume and several DMT specialist interviews have underscored this, as well as the challenges associated with adherence. Sometimes a negative mood state, a sense of hopelessness, or clinical depression will interfere with the honest desires to take care of oneself. Sometimes, to avoid negative side effects or grueling, limiting routines, patients assert control over their own experience through intentional non-adherence (Turk and Meichenbaum 1988). Therapeutic influence on adherence can have indirect but vital benefits. In my study of DMT for adults hospitalized with cystic fibrosis (CF), there appears to have been a positive effect on self-reported adherence for those who participated in the treatment (see Chapter 4, and Goodill in press). The pathways, or mechanisms, by which this came about are unknown and were not investigated. It is conceivable that the DMT brought about an increase in body awareness, and accordingly more sensitivity to bodily cues that needed self-care attention. Another possible explanation is that the supportive environment of the DMT sessions led to an increased sense of self-worth or body-esteem (Cash and Pruzinsky 1990) and this could motivate better self-care. This is pure conjecture, but points out the merit of measuring adherence as part of medical DMT clinical outcome studies. This finding also raises the question of mechanisms of DMT in the context of medical illness.

Mind/body perceptions

Patient perceptions of experiences and relationships, of one's own abilities and worth, of life remembered and life remaining, are valid indications of therapeutic effect. When subjectively felt mind/body phenomena are expressed in the patient's own words, we have important information about what the treatment (DMT or other) means to that person. And it is the meaning of the experience that is essential (Kaplan 1990; Moerman and Jonas 2002; Taylor *et al.* 2000). The distinction between pain and suffering is a prime example of this (Barsky and Baszender 1998; S. Imus, personal communication, July 12, 2002).

Consider the power of the narrative data. Serlin's patient reflects on her DMT experience and says, "It gives a spaciousness to my cells...and then it gives spaciousness to my spirit" (Serlin *et al.* 2000, p.131). A man with CF emerges from relaxation and says, "Well, if my death is anything like that maybe it won't be so bad!" The participant in Petrone's cancer support group wrote that DMT "brings a sense of lightness to a very heavy, serious illness" (Petrone 1997, pp.52–3). These people are speaking directly of integrated mind/body experiences with metaphor and sensory language. The examples provide evidence that the modality has benefits for some medically ill people. A systematic analysis of qualitative data like this could be compelling and worthwhile.

The mind/body dynamic

A DMT perspective could inform the rapidly advancing research efforts to unpack the intricacies of the mind/body interaction. Futterman's research into immunological correlates of emotional states employed method actors who could move themselves into various moods (Futterman *et al.* 1992). Similar study of movement states could explore if and how DMT interventions might correlate with immunological, cardiovascular, pulmonary or other physiological indicators of health or immune functioning (Bojner-Horwitz *et al.* 2003; Goodill 2000b). The studies by

Bernstein and Cafarelli (1972), Hunt (1973) and Sakamoto (2001) have begun this process by exploring aspects of DMT theory using electromyography as a physiologic measure. Dulicai's study (1995), which coupled LMA-based movement assessment with standardized neurological assessments, is another model for validating DMT theory about the integration of mind, brain and movement functioning.

Krantz's study (1994; Pennebaker 2000) raised useful questions about the differential contributions of nondiscursive (dance/movement) and discursive (writing) processes to the health-enhancing benefits of emotional expression. In addition, Krantz's study replicated and extended a major research theme in the larger health care field, thereby placing DMT findings in a context with other widely recognized work. We need more studies of this kind to discern the mechanisms of DMT in relation to health, and to test theories concerning the modality in general health care.

There are lingering questions about the dynamic between mood, physiology and behavior. Salovey et al. (2000) phrased it this way:

> People's behavior may be motivated by the desire to improve their mood, but the process by which behavior alters mood is unclear. Specifically, research is needed to tease apart the relative influences of physiological changes associated with the behavior and cognitive expectancies regarding the influence of the behavior on emotional experience. In addition, investigators may need to attend to a broader array of emotional states when assessing the degree to which a behavior successfully made people feel better. (para. 35)

Here, the researchers were discussing two challenges that DMT could help to address. They comment on the need to expand the question of emotional states beyond the broad categories of positive and negative emotions. Dance/movement therapists, with their expertise in eliciting and negotiating subtle changes in affect state, and well-developed theory regarding nonverbal manifestations of emotion (Chodorow 1995), could contribute well to research on this question. Second, the "influence of behavior on emotional experience" is clearly in the domain of DMT practice, where the pathways of mind/body influence have always been understood as bidirectional, and the route from behavior to emotion is commonly traveled (Levy 1988).

Two other ideas surfaced in earlier chapters of this text, and are reiterated as topics for research attention. First are the intriguing questions that Cohen (1997) raised regarding stillness and movement in relation to altered awareness and mind/body harmony (see Chapter 2). Second, Kasovac's observations (personal communication, August 9, 2000) about the development of body image in technology-dependent young children also have merit and relevance for DMT research.

Methodological considerations

The idea of the mind/body integration has brought new research questions to the surface. New questions may require different forms of inquiry. This section explores some of the research design and methodology concepts that could advance medical DMT research within the competitive health care research field.

Collaboration

Schwartz (1982) observed that in a contextual approach to research, multi-causality is considered, but even then, "disillusionment sets in as the picture becomes more complex. Competing 'single' causes are found, and so-called moderating variables are discovered that may attenuate, mask, or even at times reverse the effects of the presumed single cause" (p.1043). At this point, researchers will try:

> (a) breaking the problem into subproblems or areas – setting up new formistic categories, and thus allowing the investigator to return to Stage 1 and 2 [formistic or mechanistic models] research, (b) ignoring certain data that do not fit with the presumed primary mechanism, (c) giving up on research as being too complex, or (d) adapting an organistic-systems approach to the research... This [fourth] view makes the tasks of research and practice much more difficult because it requires that multiple variables be assessed and then integrated and interpreted. (Schwartz 1982, p.1043)

Nonetheless, to truly embrace the biopsychosocial model in clinical research, the organistic-systems approach makes sense. The only way that dance/movement therapists or any other researchers can address the multilevel, multicausal questions that are at the heart of wholistic health care is to work in multi-disciplinary teams and to think about the research in interdisciplinary ways. Therefore it is essential for the medical DMT researcher to develop strong collaborative relationships with professionals in other health care specialties. In those relationships, all parties strive to find common theoretical ground and to keep the focus on the biopsychosocial needs of the patient. This kind of collaborative research can be very creative, and can yield genuinely new insights about the mind/body integration. Serlin's research collaboration with the team at California Pacific Medical Center is a good example of successful multidisciplinary work.

Fertile possibilities for research collaboration exist in the arts arena, and are identified in a report from the 2003 Arts in Healthcare Symposium. In this meeting of leaders in the (U.S.) National Institutes of Health, the Society for Arts in Healthcare (SAH), and the National Endowment for the Arts the following areas were targeted for research: "Long-term/end of life care (arts and diabetes, cancer, Alzheimer's); Quality/cost of care, patient satisfaction; Staff job satisfaction/and burnout; Medical education/service learning; Prevention" (Palmer and Leniart 2003, p. 11). There is a good deal of overlap between these topics and the medical DMT work that has been described in earlier chapters.

Mixed methodology and single-case designs

When the research lenses are widened to take in the complexities of multicausality and contextual issues, the task can become daunting. In the "gold standard" of clinical outcomes research, the prospective randomized, placebo-controlled design, the details and richness of human experience are often lost in the volume of data that is represented numerically for inferential statistical analysis (Cassileth *et al.* 1994). On the other hand, one usually cannot make generalizations from the findings of purely qualitative research; but to endorse and fund clinical services, insurers need to know that a treatment will be effective more often than not. To exploit the merits of each approach, two research design options, mixed methodology and case study, are recommended. Each is described below.

Mixed methodology studies are designed to ask questions of both a qualitative and quantitative nature, and collect data of both types (Tashakkori and Teddlie 1998). This may be done in phases, where a qualitative study is conducted to explore and discern patterns using open-ended or process-oriented questions. This may be followed by a confirmatory phase using formal hypothesis testing and large numbers of participants, so that findings can be generalized. Another option is to combine both approaches in the same study, so that the two types of data confirm impressions from each other. This model can retain the richness and nuance of real and lived experience, while providing clear information about the effectiveness of a treatment program. For all of these reasons, blending qualitative and quantitative methods is recommended for complementary and alternative therapy research (Cassidy *et al.* 1994). At this juncture, the blend is quite appropriate for research on DMT in medical care because both types of questions are pressing.

Our study of acupuncture for women with polycystic ovarian syndrome (PCOS) (Newman *et al.* 2000) is an example of both multidisciplinary research and mixed methodology. The team consisted of a family physician, two health psychologists, a medical student assistant, a dance/movement therapist, an obstetrician-gynecologist also trained as a medical acupuncturist and a reproductive endocrinologist. The research questions included: "What is the experience of women undergoing acupuncture for anovulation?" (qualitative inquiry) and "Does acupuncture work to bring about ovulation for women with PCOS?" (quantitative focus). Data analysis was a collaborative group effort to gradually piece together the different types of data and form a new synthesis of information.

The study of DMT for older adults with neurological insult (Berrol *et al.* 1997) is another good example of mixed method research. Data from standardized instruments, video analysis, participant interviews, therapist field notes and formal movement assessment converged in a coherent picture of how DMT benefits this population. The Dibbel-Hope study (2000) did the same, with standardized instruments, participant interviews and therapists' impressions. Integrated analysis and convergence of different data types can reconcile apparent discrepancies in data and provide realistic, relevant findings.

Case study is recommended for new research questions (Chaiklin 2000) and for disciplines in the complementary and alternative therapies (Aldridge 1994; Lukoff, Edwards and Miller 1998) such as DMT. Case study is receiving attention as a powerful yet flexible design for clinical research in mainstream fields such as psychology (Kazdin 1982; Morgan and Morgan 2001). Findings from a single case study using experimental methods (with baseline phases for collecting control data, and well-defined treatment phases) can make treatment effects clear. "A causal relation between the intervention and performance on the dependent measures is demonstrated if each behavior (individual or situation) changes when (and only when) the program is introduced" (Kazdin 1982, p.478). The case study is ideal for the common situation where one form of treatment cannot be isolated from the milieu or total program, and where this would constitute a "multiple treatment confound" in controlled group research designs (Stewart, McMullen and Rubin 1994). Each medical patient is unique unto him- or herself, and the course of most medical conditions can be only conservatively predicted. The case study can preserve that uniqueness, and welcomes information about family, school, work, religious, medical and physiological aspects of the patient's life. The findings cannot be generalized to the population from which the case is drawn, however "case studies occasionally have had remarkable impact when several cases were accumulated. Although each case is studied individually, the information is accumulated to identify more general relationships" (Kazdin 1982, p.8).

Standardization of treatment

Standardization of treatment is one technique for demonstrating the effectiveness of a clinical modality. To standardize the intervention is to ensure that the method being tested is reliably similar across patients, patient groups, settings, and therapists delivering the treatment. However, for treatment approaches based in experiential, interactional, improvisational and creative processes, restricting sessions to a prescribed sequence of events can actually compromise a study's validity. Serlin discussed the issue as follows, in relation to the existential approach to group therapy that was studied in the collaborative research with breast cancer patients:

> This existential base is important, because as the alternative and complementary health movement spreads, there is a push to make all interventions standardized and manualized. Standardizing an intervention has the advantage of allowing for comparative research, and for training health professionals to repeat the program in new locations. An existentially-based group takes issue with this form of standardization, however, since it is based on the principle that the imagery and material arise from the participants and the group itself, and are not imposed by an "authority". (Serlin *et al.* 2000, p.129)

To alter the methods and style with which a therapy is usually conducted in order to study its effectiveness is in fact a source of bias in the research (Cassidy *et al.* 1994). It has been suggested that "interference with normal spontaneity and flexibility in patient–therapist interactions" be avoided or at the least, noted in the study report (Cassidy *et al.* 1994, p.346).

The challenge lies in the fact that for potential funders of medical DMT research, it is important to describe the intervention in as much detail and consistency as possible. What might be best is to standardize and describe the overall clinical approach, including the basic structure of sessions, the salient themes that are expected to be addressed, and give examples of possible clinical scenarios. If the treatment program is designed in phases, these can be predictably described. In the case of multiple clinicians providing intervention, this establishes sufficient consistency across providers. The Berrol *et al.* (1997) study followed this procedure. In addition, a research proposal or report should clarify the process orientation of the intervention and explain why the retention of this element is important to the effectiveness of the treatment.

Systematic therapeutic learning

Cassileth and colleagues (1994) identified DMT as one of the complementary therapies that involves systematic therapeutic learning. This means that the therapy involves a learning process, and that with experience the patient or client gradually becomes more adept with the clinical method. Presumably then, the effectiveness of the therapy will be mediated by the amount of exposure the patient or study participants have had to DMT. The authors advised that study participants in clinical outcome research achieve a basic level of learning in the modality and that studies control for the amount of learning among participants. This is potentially relevant to all research on DMT's effectiveness.

Psychophysiological measurement

From psychoneuroimmunology (PNI) and other work that combines psychological and biological data, we have compelling evidence for the mind/body integration, the bidirectionality of the relationship, neurohormonal processes, and the effect of emotions on disease and health (see Chapters 2 and 3). Taken together, the findings undergird DMT theory in exciting ways. Indeed, neuroscience may ultimately explain how DMT processes work (Berrol 1992), but there are a number of methodological issues to consider in any work that may attempt this.

Most psychophysiological measurement is best conducted with study participants who are nearly immobile and this limit in current technology has influenced psychophysiological measurement coming out of the DMT field. Electromyography (EMG) is used in biomechanics and kinesiology research to document the innervation of muscles and quantify muscle activity (McDonough 2001). A handful of studies have employed EMG for DMT and related research despite this limitation. For example, Bernstein and Cafarelli's study (1972) measured Effort production in the muscles of the subject's right arm alone. More recently, in Sakamoto's study (2001), the range of movement was necessarily restricted in order not to disrupt the EMG instruments. Chatfield (1998) used this method to explore questions related to habitual neuromuscular patterns and movement initiation in dance sequences, with movement restricted to a forward pushing of the hand. While electroencephalogram (EEG) measurement would yield rich and fascinating data concerning brain functioning during expressive movement, the current technology available to the average neuroscience researcher does not permit clear EEG measurement while a subject moves the head (Field et al. 1998; Scott Bunce, PhD, neuropsychology researcher, personal communication, September 13, 2001).

Mobile EMG battery packs are now available to measure muscle activity in more active people, but these systems are easily overwhelmed by the complexity and volume of movement that occurs during spontaneous, full body dance/ movement activity (A. Karduna, movement scientist, personal communication,

August 14, 1998). Three-dimensional spatial pathways in human movement can now be digitalized using kinematic methods. Using kinematics, Streepay and Gross (1998) found that dancers' emotional intent (for fear, anger and neutral emotion) could be differentiated through this detailed, quantitated portrait of movement dynamics. Lotan and Yirmiya (2002) used kinematic methods and elements of the Kestenberg Movement Profile to study the body movement of toddlers in the process of falling asleep.

Movement involves SNS arousal, and as explained earlier, there are hormonal and possibly immunologic sequelae to a sympathetically aroused state. Futterman noted that her subjects' movement confounded data associated with SNS activation, and may have produced some of the variability in immune system parameters (Futterman *et al.* 1992). In addition, patterns of hormone production and release follow circadian rhythms (Sherwood 1997) and are also affected by food intake.

In PNI reactivity studies, a subject is given or presented with some kind of environmental, emotional or chemical challenge to the neuroendocrine or immune system (IS) and researchers then track the responses. Cohen's study (1991) is a good example. He presented allergic patients with a ragweed-pollen challenge, and then measured the response of the IS to either a guided imagery intervention or no intervention (the control group).

Researchers should be aware that there is a time lag between the introduction of a stimulus and the measurable responses of the body's homeostatic systems. The autonomic nervous system (ANS) responds within seconds to minutes; organ responses to stressors will occur within minutes to hours; innate immune responses are made within hours, and adaptive immunity develops over days to weeks. Components of the immune system activate within minutes, hours, days and weeks (Parham 2000; Rossi 1993). In addition, the various methods for obtaining biological samples are also time sensitive. The hormone cortisol, commonly sampled as an indicator of stress levels, can be measured in the blood, the saliva and in urine (Field *et al.* 1992). Elevated levels of cortisol can be detected 20–30 minutes after the onset of stress (Field *et al.* 1998; Rabin *et al.* 1994; Schneiderman and McCabe 1989). Some immune system samples can be taken in as little as a half hour after a stressor is introduced (Keller *et al.* 1994).

Selecting relevant immunological measures is critical and selecting the most appropriate way of analyzing samples is also important. In PNI, the analysis of samples for immune system components is called an *assay*. Kiecolt-Glaser and Glaser (1992) recommended taking not one but several immune measures in a study and analyzing the activity of those components rather than simply their numbers. They cautioned, "No single assay or group of assays provides a standard, global measure of immune function... In general, qualitative or functional assays appear to be more sensitive to psychosocial stressors than quantitative assays." (Kiecolt-Glaser and Glaser 1992, p.569). Other researchers have agreed that no single measure of immunity can fully represent the competence of the immune system (Jemmott and McClelland 1989).

Secretory Immunoglobulin A (S-IgA) is a popular indicator of IS activity (Burns 1996; Goff *et al.* 1997; Simon 1991). Like cortisol, it can be sampled from saliva. Secretory IgA prevents infectious agents from adhering to mucosal body surfaces and invading the body's barriers. This glycoprotein is attractive to the researcher who wishes to avoid inducing experimental stress in a blood-draw procedure. However, the techniques for using S-IgA are controversial. Some authorities have argued for the measurement of only S-IgA antibodies produced in response to an antigen challenge (Stone *et al.* 1987) and others have maintained that total concentration levels of whole saliva provide a more complete, and therefore better, picture of immune system activity via S-IgA (Jemmott and McClelland 1989). PNI researchers use both methods, but either way salivary flow rate should be taken into consideration when analyzing either aspect of salivary IgA. Flow rate fluctuates with ANS activity and this alters concentration levels in ways that may not be related to the research question.

Because the body's homeostatic systems are exquisitely responsive to changes in the internal and external environment, most of the parameters of interest when studying the mind/body interaction are influenced by multiple events at any given moment. Researchers who attempt to describe the effects of one such event or stimulus (for example, the postural expression of anger or the receipt of a warm hug) should attempt to control for the unrelated variables that would obfuscate the desired data. Researchers have cautioned that PNI studies should control for the following variables: drugs and medications, alcohol and caffeine intake, acute and chronic health patterns, changes in sleep patterns or in weight, and cigarette smoking (Glaser and Kiecolt-Glaser 1998). Studies including the measurement of ANS activity should control for exercise patterns, excessive heat or cold, levels of distress, and personality type (Schneiderman and McCabe 1989). For managing these unwieldy variables, Schneiderman and McCabe suggest a logical strategy of taking thorough baseline control measures before introducing the phenomenon under study.

The opinions and ideas presented in this chapter grew primarily out of this author's research and clinical experience. Others may have different and quite valid perspectives, and will surely generate countless other valuable research foci for medical DMT. Medical DMT is generally practiced in the complex and fast-paced world of health care. The health care field is richly endowed with brilliant researchers and clinicians eager to discover new and effective treatment methods. Creative collaborations with scientifically prepared colleagues will enable dance/movement therapists to participate in these discussions.

CHAPTER 8

Patient–Provider Communication: Implications for Dance/ Movement Therapy

Earlier chapters in this volume describe the importance of social support from spouses, family members, friends, community networks and support groups or therapy. The nature of the relationships between patients and their health care providers also impacts the quality of care. Patient–provider communication, a component of these relationships, is increasingly recognized as a key factor in all health care contexts and has been linked to the effectiveness of treatment and better patient coping (Farber 2002). Interest in the topic has burgeoned in the past 15 years. A search of electronic research databases on the topic will yield literally hundreds of articles from the disciplines of nursing, medicine, psychology and other allied therapies, with a large proportion from nursing, psychology and the social sciences, and most since 1985.

This chapter includes a brief review of the literature on the patient–provider relationship, communication and the role of nonverbal factors. Nonverbal communication research is fundamental to the practice and principles of dance/ movement therapy (DMT), and the field has a particular relevance to understanding the nonverbal dimensions of patient–provider communication and clinical relationships. In addition, DMT concepts and clinical techniques may be adapted to enhance the communication between health care providers and their patients, specifically through education and training activities.

Warner's (1985) comprehensive review of the research on patient–provider communication outlined three primary types of studies used:

- *correlational studies* wherein patients' self-reports on satisfaction, adherence, and impressions of the relationship are compared to observed elements of the interaction with provider

- *pre-test–post-test* studies wherein health care providers in training are taught about communication and tested regarding knowledge, attitudes or acquisition of specific skills

- *experimental studies* wherein a communication intervention is given to one group of patients and outcome is compared to a control group (Warner 1985, p.46).

The proposed link with DMT assessment and clinical techniques is with the first two of these three types.

Across the spectrum of literature, communication is acknowledged as important. The quality of the clinical relationship and the effectiveness of communication in it have been linked with patient satisfaction, adherence and medical outcomes. However, it is not yet clear exactly how this factor interacts with other major influences such as disease severity, features of the treatment regimen, financial resources and the premorbid emotional state of the patient (Warner 1985). An impressive body of research by Robin DiMatteo and colleagues led her to state that, "the physician–patient relationship is at the heart of patient nonadherence and that to solve the problem, communication between doctors and patients must be improved" (DiMatteo 1995, p.211).

Studies from medicine, nursing and psychology

In one study on patient satisfaction with hospital services, attributes of caring and empathy emerged as two of twelve critical dimensions (Bowers, Swan and Koehler 1994). The researchers combined focus group methodology with a questionnaire about patients' experiences in the hospital (N = 298 for the questionnaire arm of the study) (Bowers *et al.*, para. 15). From the focus groups, they learned that caring was understood as a level of involvement beyond courtesy and responsiveness, or understanding the patient. Rather, caring "implies a personal, human involvement…with emotions approaching love for the patient" (para. 13). The researchers concluded, "Patients define health care quality in terms of empathy, reliability, responsiveness, communication and caring. These are human dimensions related to how the health care service was delivered, not the technical competence of the provider" (para.15). Even though this study was conducted from a health care management and marketing perspective, the findings recall the tenets of the wholism described in Chapter 1 of this volume, and invite a biopsychosocial approach.

A study of patient–physician communication in palliative care treatment visits revealed that oncologists who had positive attitudes toward psychosocial and emotional functioning, and believed it to be important, spent more time discussing these issues with their patients (Detmar *et al.* 2001). The researchers also noted that perceived time pressure, a common complaint of both doctors and patients, tends to interfere with the exchange of information. Using analysis of audio-recordings, they found that emotional problems were more likely to be discussed in appointments that began when scheduled, as opposed to those delayed.

Smith (2001) argued well for more patient-centered interviewing during medical visits. He proposed a clear and feasible five-step interviewing method that puts the physician in a receptive listening mode for the first three to five minutes of an appointment, before shifting to the doctor-centered process that is more focused on details of the disease and specific intervention planning. According to Smith, patient-centered interviewing "encourages the expression of the patient's personal thoughts and feelings, and the healing impact that attends this expression" (Smith 2001, p.31). The procedure instructs the provider to use verbal and nonverbal behaviors that resemble techniques in supportive psychotherapy. For example, the following appear in "Step 3: Nonfocused interviewing."

2. 'Nonfocusing' open-ended skills should be used: silence, neutral utterances, nonverbal encouragement.

3. 'Focusing' in an open-ended way is appropriate if one needs to get the patient talking. Examples are: echoing, summarising and making requests...

5. The provider should obtain additional data from the following sources: nonverbal cues, physical characteristics, autonomic changes, accoutrements and environment. (Smith 2001, p.32)

And from "Step 4: Focused interviewing:"

2. Extend the story to the psychosocial context of the symptoms.

3. Develop a free flow of personal data.

4. Develop an emotional focus.

5. Address the emotion(s). (Smith 2001, p.32)

A series of studies on Smith's patient-centered interviewing method demonstrated that the approach can be learned by medical students and residents, nursing students, nurses and physician assistants. It may lead to decreased somatic complaints and social dysfunction and increased satisfaction with care for patients of medical residents trained in the method (Smith 2001, p.33).

The dynamics of touch permeate health care. Medical patients in both inpatient and outpatient settings are routinely touched and moved by workers ranging from physicians to nurses to phlebotomists, and therapists of all kinds. Hospital staffing patterns often place nurses on longer but fewer shifts, and the use of hospitalist physicians puts patients in the care of physicians they have not met until coming into the hospital. This means that most in-hospital patient–provider touch occurs between relative strangers. Research on touch has identified gender differences in the response to touch among patients in the hospital. Women who were touched on the hand by the nurse during an educational interaction at the bedside responded more favorably than did men who received the same touch (Whitcher and Fisher 1979, as cited in Warner 1985). The patient's interpretation of touch is influenced by the amount of touch, the gender of the touching professional, values and current emotional state (Farber, Novack and O'Brien 1997). These many nuances suggest that the development of touch skills should be included in professional preparation of health care workers.

Farber *et al.* (1997) explored the question of interpersonal boundaries in the doctor–patient relationship, recommending that doctors can form "empathic yet objective" relationships with their patients (Farber *et al.* 1997, p.2291); that they can "find a connection with their patients, yet prevent enmeshment from occurring" (Farber *et al.* 1997, p.2294). And they included kinesthetic aspects of the relationship in the discussion: "Boundary parameters include the contact time between the 2 individuals, the amount of information shared by the patient and the physician, the degree of shared decision making, and *the shared physical and emotional space* [italics added]" (Farber *et al.* 1997, p.2292). When physicians consider the shared physical and emotional space in this way, an interdisciplinary dialogue is opened up, and it becomes possible to explore concepts germane to DMT and the other body-based therapies, such as intersubjectivity and somatic countertransference (Pallaro 1994).

Trust is a vital component of all helping relationships. In health care, the helping relationship is extended to the family and loved ones of a patient. A good portion of the medical DMT work described in this volume involves the dance/movement therapist establishing relationships with families. Indeed, all providers do this, although nursing has given the topic of trust the most research attention. Through a concept analysis, Lynn-McHale and Deatrick (2000) identified six characteristics of trust in the relationships between patients' family members and health care providers. They described this particular manifestation of trust as "a *process*, consisting of *varying levels*, that *evolves over time* and is based on *mutual intention, reciprocity*, and *expectations* [italics added]" (Lynn-McHale and Deatrick 2000, para. 1). Good communication was identified as one precondition to trust, and active listening as a component of communication. Active listening is a constellation of nonverbal behaviors, and so the researchers implicitly addressed nonverbal phenomena in communication. The data used for the concept analysis were samples from the literature, but the notion of trust as a process evolving over time with reciprocity is strikingly similar to the way dance/movement therapists view the movement-based relationship-building process in this specialty (Schmais 1974).

Warner discussed the importance of congruence between nonverbal messages such as facial expression, gaze, touch, interpersonal distance, vocal tone and body movement, and verbal information in health care, noting that "through attention to these nonverbal cues, particularly when they are discrepant with the verbal messages, a medical practitioner may acquire valuable information about the patient's emotional state" (Warner 1985, p.52). Knapp and Hall (1997) underscored the necessity to embrace and integrate both in research on human communication:

> Ray Birdwhistell, a pioneer in nonverbal research, reportedly said that studying only *nonverbal* communication is like studying *noncardiac* physiology... The verbal dimension is so intimately woven and subtly represented in so much of what has been previously labeled *non*verbal that the term does not always adequately describe the behavior under study. (Knapp and Hall 1997, p.11)

DiMatteo, who worked with Robert Rosenthal on the PONS (Profile of Nonverbal Sensitivity) test, has made significant contributions to the body of knowledge regarding nonverbal aspects of patient–provider communication. The PONS is widely employed as a reliable and valid measure of one's ability to (a) encode or send nonverbal messages that are consistent with one's intent, and (b) decode or read messages sent by others (Knapp and Hall 1997). The content of such messages may convey information about emotions, attitudes, needs, status or, as the kinesics researchers noted, they may maintain the social order (Scheflen with Scheflen 1972). Individual tendencies towards good encoding or good decoding may be formed early by experiences in the family of origin (Knapp and Hall 1997), but the skills can be taught and mastered.

Aptly, much of the work by DiMatteo and her colleagues has focused on physicians. Even though patients experience many different providers in the system and other important care relationships develop, the physician–patient relationship is where most decision making takes place and where most patients direct their trust. Their research program has aimed to address the "dearth of information about what goes on between physicians and patients on a nonverbal level" (DiMatteo, Hays and Prince 1986, p.592). In several of their studies, the PONS has been used to measure physicians' abilities to encode nonverbal expression of emotions and decode the patient's nonverbal communications. They have linked both skills to patient satisfaction (DiMatteo *et al.* 1986). Most medical training on nonverbal communication focuses on the doctor's ability to read the patient's nonverbal cues as part of assessment. In one study, the researchers filmed medical residents posing several different expressions because (a) "physicians are required frequently to control or pose emotions to communicate empathic understanding to their patients" and (b) "large positive and significant correlations have been found between posed encoding and spontaneous expressiveness" (DiMatteo *et al.* 1986, p.585). The better encoders had patients who were more satisfied with their care, and they also had heavier workloads. In this study, physician workload was used as one indicator of patient satisfaction, based on the premise that the larger the caseload the more adherent patients are with appointment making and keeping. The researchers identified several potentially confounding variables, but recommended that future work should "provide a precise understanding of the workings of nonverbal communication in health care" (DiMatteo *et al.* 1986, p.592).

With the notable exceptions of the work described above, much of the published medical work to date minimizes the nonverbal dimension in a few discernable ways. First, in most studies nonverbal communication (NVC) is addressed as an afterthought, or as only one component in a sea of verbal language skills. Second, when NVC is addressed, the terminology tends to be rudimentary and imprecise, especially when compared to the detailed level of description used in DMT (Schonwetter, Hawke and Knight 1999). Third, when professional training programs in health care communication are described, the NVC is usually addressed as something the provider is observing in the patient for information-gathering purposes. This approach ignores substantial research on the mutual nature of nonverbal communication (Condon 1968; Condon and Ogston 1969; Davis and Hadiks 1994; Scheflen 1982), which would place equal emphasis on the provider's movement behavior. These three deficits in the mainstream literature on NVC in health care indicate a role for the dance/movement therapist in research and provider education.

Research from a DMT perspective

Fraenkel (1986) conducted a study of interaction between medical residents and their patients using two kinds of shared behavior events, synchrony and echoing, to assess the role of the nonverbal dimension in the exchange of information during medical consultations. Specifically, she explored the "relationships among dyadic nonverbal behaviors, varying levels of empathy, patient satisfaction, and patient comprehension and retention of doctor-offered information" (Fraenkel, 1986, p.61). The Fraenkel-Franks Index of Shared Behaviors (FFISB) was developed and used to capture incidences of synchrony (when movements by both participants begin and end simultaneously and move at the same rate) and echoing (when there is a delay between the onset of the first movement and that of the second) in paired movement during dyadic interaction (Fraenkel 1986, p.74). Fraenkel's data revealed a positive correlation between synchronous behavior and the patient's accurate recollection of doctor-offered information, but no such correlation emerged for echoing or neutral nonverbal interaction. The implications of this are important on two levels. First, if a patient is to adhere to medical advice or prescripted self-care regimens, he or she has to be able to remember the doctor's instructions. Thus, there are implications for adherence. Second, the data suggest that nonverbal interaction has an immediate relationship to cognitive aspects of patient care. The moment of synchrony is at once a cognitive and motoric event co-occurring for both participants. This study is an excellent example of research that attends to the congruence of verbal and nonverbal behaviors.

To explore the potential impact of shared behaviors in a particular alternative medicine modality, acupuncture, we studied the frequency of synchrony and echoing behaviors between a physician-acupuncturist and five female patients. All the women were diagnosed with polycystic ovarian syndrome (PCOS) and were participants in a multiple baseline case study of acupuncture for the treatment of anovulation, which is one component of that syndrome (Newman *et al.* 2000). The instrument used to measure shared nonverbal behaviors was a modified version of Fraenkel's FFISB that was altered in two ways for this study. First, parameters for "quality synchrony" and "quality echoing" were added. Here, quality refers to the predominant Effort quality observed in the movement (see Laban 1980). Second, the assignment of an "echo" score was given to the second mover in an echoing sequence, following the logic that it is the second movement that creates an echo. A ten-minute verbal discussion between the acupuncturist and the patient preceded each of twelve weekly acupuncture sessions, and three of these discussions were videotaped (near the beginning, middle and end of the treatment phase). Two trained raters scored thirteen video segments on five types of synchrony (exact, approximate, spatial, quality and rhythmic) and the same five types of echoing. Rater agreement was assessed at 0.97 using a sampling of the 114 minutes scored and a frequency ratio of that sample (Kazdin 1982; R. Cruz, personal communication, October 2000). Consistent with Fraenkel's findings

(1986) we observed far more echoing than synchrony in this doctor–patient interaction. Data analysis tracked the frequency of total echoing across time, and frequencies were interpreted in relation to theories of nonverbal rapport and relationship building (Goodill 2000a). In all five treatment sequences, the doctor echoed the patient more frequently in the beginning of the relationship. This represents the doctor's attempts to build rapport and trust, a phenomenon described in the DMT literature and elsewhere (Davis and Hadicks 1994). In four of the five dyads, we saw the ratio of doctor-echoing-patient and patient- echoing-doctor events either equalize or reverse as the treatment progressed. Echoing is a form of nonverbal reciprocity, and the data suggested to us that mutuality had evolved (in cases of equalized echoing patterns) or that the patient had developed some trust in the doctor (when later patterns showed the patient "following" the doctor more). In addition, raters recorded different types of shared movement events in each dyad, suggesting that the clinician modified her own nonverbal style to that of her patients. In-depth interviews with participants at the same measurement points confirmed this impression of their subjective experiences in the therapeutic relationship, and described the clinician as warm and caring. From a mind/body integration and PNI standpoint, it is notable that the same four women for whom we saw the echoing pattern equalize or change, all experienced either a regulation of menses, one or more ovulatory cycles or (in one case) pregnancy, during the study. The study sample was too small to infer any causal relationship between acupuncture, the quality of the relationship, its nonverbal elements, and reproductive functioning, but this case-based evidence should compel future research into these potential interactions.

Reciprocity in nonverbal exchanges may be linked to expectation. As the reader will recall from discussions of the placebo effect in Chapter 2, expectation is hypothesized to impact the effectiveness of both conventional and complementary medical therapies (Turner *et al.* 1994). Knapp and Hall (1997) offered this summary of the literature on the topic:

> We tend to reciprocate or match another's nonverbal behavior when it is perceived as generally congruent with our expectations and involvement preferences. We tend to compensate or offset another's nonverbal behavior when it is perceived as a major violation of our expectations and preferences. (p.451)

If shared expectations and the related attribute of mutual interest underlie nonverbal reciprocity, then new questions arise as to how the nonverbal dynamic, as a non-specific effect, might moderate treatment outcomes.

Proposals for DMT contributions to NVC research and training in health care

DMT methods used to assess interaction include observation of shared postures and gestures (Davis and Hadiks 1990, 1994; Navarre 1982), accommodation of body shapes (Dulicai 1977; Loman and Foley 1996) and touch patterns, echoing and synchrony (Fraenkel 1983, 1986), rhythmic and other aspects of attunement (Amighi *et al.* 1999; Kestenberg 1975) and reciprocity (Stern 1977). DMT assessment strategies have long integrated the concept of co-action, which, according to Scheflen (1982), sees the model of "the opera or the theater or of orchestra" as a better metaphor for communication than, say, the tennis match (Scheflen 1982, p.20). In addition, the commonly employed concepts of self-synchrony and interactional synchrony, articulated by Condon and colleagues (Condon 1968; Condon and Ogston 1969) and linguistic-kinesic research by Birdwhistell (1970), Scheflen and Scheflen (1972) and others, are based on integrated analyses of verbal and nonverbal content. These contributors have informed assessment and treatment in DMT since its inception as a psychotherapeutic modality (Levy 1988). The discussion to follow highlights findings that could be relevant in provider–patient communication.

Consider the problem of time pressure. The perception of time pressure, a sense of urgency, is displayed in movement behavior (North 1972). Modulation of the Effort quality *quickness* towards more use of *sustainment* can change the feel of an interaction without actually increasing the duration of the exchange.

Fraenkel (1983) investigated the way that echoing and synchrony contribute to empathy and rapport in dyadic exchanges. Echoing, she learned, and not synchrony seemed to accompany the process of building empathy. Synchrony may indicate a kind of "ultra-empathy" (Fraenkel 1983, p.43) with implications for psychotherapy and, as described above with medical residents, successful health care communications. Rhythmic synchrony is a form of interpersonal attunement learned in the original relationship between infant and caregiver (usually a mothering figure) (Kestenberg 1975). Thus, the template for joining another temporally is embedded in deep neurophysiologic processes (Berrol 1992; Condon 1968; Condon and Ogston 1969) and available to all mentally and physically healthy adults. Echoing also has its roots in early life, in the intricate dance that mothers and infants perform with facial cues, vocalizations, turn-taking and touch (Stern 1977). This acuity with nonverbal reciprocity is a substrate of all human interaction. It needs only to be brought into awareness and understood as important.

Navarre (1982) showed that when interactants shared postures (i.e., "mirrored" each other with shared positions in space and used similar dynamic movement qualities), they reported more positive assessments of themselves and the other participant, and assessed themselves as similar to the other participant in the dyad. Interestingly, the strength of the correlation between posture sharing and positive feelings in the interaction was moderated by the movement quality (Efforts) observed in the postural adjustments and other movement. Specifically, when the research assistant reflected only position in space but not Effort quality, subjects rated themselves positively but not the interviewer, and did not rate the interviewer as friendly (Navarre 1982, p.37). Dance/movement therapists are unique in the health care system in their ability to observe and intervene at the nuanced level of the Effort repertoire. Navarre's findings suggest that movement-focused education of health care professionals, attending to both posture and movement quality, could improve the subjective experiences of patient–provider interactions. The basic DMT clinical methods of "reflect and respond" (Sandel 1993b) could inform such training.

Impasses in medical decision making often are the result of poor communication between doctors and patients or their family members (Perrin 2001). With the assessment skills listed here, medical dance/movement therapists could easily analyze the communication patterns and make recommendations towards more sensitive and attuned interactions. There is evidence that training programs aimed at improving physicians' communication skills can work (Detmar *et al.* 2001), and this may apply to nonverbal skills as well. In the study by DiMatteo *et al.* (1986), physicians who scored higher in affective encoding also scored higher on the Affective Communication Test (ACT), a self-report instrument in which respondents describe their own nonverbal emotional expression. Those with acting experience also tend to score higher on the ACT than those without such experience (Friedman *et al.* 1980, as cited in DiMatteo *et al.* 1986). This would suggest that training aimed at enhancing nonverbal emotional expressivity may be effective in improving those skills.

Finally, DMT offers a vehicle for developing creativity. Rodenhauser (1996) observed, "As medicine becomes more scientific and technological, questions about the ways in which the practice of medicine can be enriched through the cultivation of creativity become more compelling" (p.6). He asked, "Should not the medical education process include cultivation of creativity?" (p.2). Dossey (2001), a leader in mind/body medicine, stated that patients need physicians who have learned to balance intellect with feeling and reason with intuition. "To achieve balance, however," he wrote, "we must create something that has been missing in healthcare: a space for the nonrational, intuitive side of the mind" (Dossey 2001, p.5). DMT and other Creative Arts Therapies (CAT) techniques create such a space and cultivate the creative impulse, and should be included in consultative or educational designs for medical professionals.

This is a potent area for the development of DMT curricula. Dance/movement therapists working in medical settings could develop training modules for preservice and in-service programming. Audiences could ostensibly include any health care professionals who interact with patients and their families.

CHAPTER 9

Professional Preparation for Medical Dance/Movement Therapy

Medical application of dance/movement therapy (DMT) requires additional preparation of the dance/movement therapist who wishes to work in this area. This chapter includes recommendations for additional coursework or certifications that practitioners may need, suggestions for personal preparation, and a series of training exercises for experiential learning. The chapter will also include recommendations for approaching traditional health care systems with a complementary therapy such as DMT and forming productive collegial relationships within the health care system. These learning experiences are intended to augment basic Master's level education for DMT, not to replace it. Recommendations are derived from interviews with and published works by the many clinicians who have made this their focus, and from my own experience as a clinician, educator and researcher.

Academic preparation

Ideally, a program of courses and workshops could be offered to the dance/movement therapist who wants to specialize in medical applications. As of this writing, no such program of formal education exists specifically for the DMT specialty, and so the therapist is advised to seek and gather the following academic information independently. Much of this can be obtained through continuing education courses. To access appropriate learning opportunities, the therapist can join professional societies and associations of like-minded clinicians (see Appendix A for a list of these). If working in a hospital or medical setting, conferences, symposia and Grand Rounds comprise another type of learning venue.

The following list comprises areas of medical knowledge that the medical dance/movement therapist may need to acquire through didactic learning:

1.   Human physiology.

2.   Cardiopulmonary resuscitation training (CPR). This is usually available as in-service or continuing education training or through the Red Cross in various community settings.

3.   Bereavement counseling, including information on spiritual issues, death and dying.

4.   Readings about the psychosocial research into the condition of concern.

5.   Medical terminology for the treatments, and side effects of treatments, for the condition of concern.

The body of medical knowledge is vast, and it is realistic to concentrate at first only on the medical information on treatments, side effects and psychosocial issues related to the cluster or class of conditions that are the focus of one's clinical work.

As of this writing, the mainstream health care system is more familiar with some of the other mind/body methods. Throughout this volume, examples of research and clinical use of techniques from yoga, massage, hypnosis, meditation, Child Life therapy and martial arts forms have been cited. It is advisable for the dance/movement therapist to add one or another of these approaches to his or her clinical repertoire. The choice of which will depend on the needs of the intended clinical population and the therapist's own philosophies and proclivities. Certification is available and required for some or all of these related disciplines. Dance/movement therapists are ethically responsible for practicing only in clinical methods for which they have been prepared, and so should seek proper training and credentials for any additional modality that will be integrated into their services.

The delivery and use of relaxation techniques are currently not regulated for any health care professional group, nor is there any formal training for these useful and beneficial methods. Indeed, human service workers in almost all mental health specialties can and do offer relaxation on a regular or occasional basis. Dance/movement therapists working with medically involved people would do well to add these methods to their clinical repertoire. In the context of medical DMT, relaxation may be included for the following purposes:

1.   To provide a pleasant experience in the body, devoid of the frustrations or pain that may accompany movement when the body is impaired.

2.   As a bridge to guided imagery work.

3.   To bring to the surface imagery that may then be developed in movement structures.

4.   To help the patient develop skills of conscious body perception and energy modulation.

5.   At the end of a session, to provide for a period of constructive stillness, when sensations, images, interactions or movements experienced in the session can be quietly reviewed and integrated.

Personal preparation

Many medical DMT specialists have been drawn to their work through direct exposure to the psychosocial aspects of illness, either their own or that of loved ones. However, one needs not to have endured the challenges or tragedies of medical illness to be effective in this application. As a method actor searches within his or her own experience for an authentic emotional expression, so the healthy therapist who works with the medically ill needs to mine personal history as a source of empathy with patients. An exercise like the guided imagery of childhood illness task (see later in this chapter) can facilitate this, if only by using memories of normal childhood illness. It is recommended that we tap into our own sources of knowledge about several aspects of the work: loss, pain, death, hate, spiritual perspectives and our human relationship to the condition or illness that is the focus of the work. There may be differences in the intensity, scope, scale or stability of the problems that we share with our patients, but all of these phenomena are experienced in the course of a normal life.

Issues of loss are relevant to changes in functioning: loss through the death of loved ones, and the loss of a future as is the case in terminal illness. Loss of functioning may be temporary or permanent and may or may not include the loss of a body part or organ. This is an element of almost every chronic or life-threatening illness. Most therapists have some personal familiarity with temporary loss of physical functioning. Examination of one's feelings, responses and adaptations to that loss can be a source of information about what the patients' subjective experiences might be. As dancers, dance/movement therapists, who have derived enjoyment, recognition and a career through refined and optimal functioning of the body, may find this issue particularly threatening (Perowsky 1991).

Perowsky's self-study explored the impact of a therapist's injury and temporary impairment on the DMT process. She wrote, "My injured body reminded me of reality," and that it helped her construct a more realistic professional self-image (Perowsky 1991, p.53). Training exercises like the dancing with limitations task (see later in this chapter) can briefly replicate the experience she described. Perowsky also discussed the culture of pain and persistence in the dance world, and observed how this translated into her experience as a patient: she first tried to "tough it out," work despite pain and deny the body messages that were telling her to slow down. Imus (personal communication, July 12, 2002) observed a similar set of underlying assumptions in the chronic pain syndrome, and suggested that a cultural worldview that values struggle may contribute to the problem. In fact, Imus mused, a culture of suffering seems to inform some psychotherapy theories, and is often observed as part of the Judeo-Christian religious value system as well. These factors may also be present in the backgrounds of dance/movement therapists and taken together may influence the therapist's perspectives and attitudes. Thus, for body-oriented therapists working with people who are in pain, this warrants exploration at a personal level.

Loss also occurs through death – the permanent and complete loss of a person from one's life. As noted in the discussions of bereavement workshops (Chapter 6), therapists are confronted with this issue in their work quite frequently. Bunney (personal communication, July 15, 2002) recommends that in addition to formal bereavement counseling, therapists spend time examining their own relationships to death: including experiences with dying people, one's personal losses to death, and one's fear of death. Bunney suggests putting the issues of loss and death in a broad human perspective that may include spirituality. Deihl's work with dying patients in hospice care (personal communication, July 22, 2002) brings these issues to the center of the therapy, and requires that the therapist be able to address them directly. Death is almost always a frightening and overwhelming part of life. That's why hospice care and bereavement programs exist. To understand one's fears, to bring one's memories (perhaps even traumatic or painful) about death to the surface, and to integrate these with a professional role identification, equips the therapist working with medical populations with an essential tool. Deihl describes how the hospice therapist helps the family "demystify" death. In order to do that the therapist needs to demystify the process for him- or herself first.

Spirituality may or may not involve formal participation in an organized religion. The benefits of a spiritual perspective have been described from health and mental health standpoints, in relation to the terminally ill and those coping with chronic illness (Horrigan 2000; McCollough *et al.* 2000). It is, of course, the patient's spiritual life or religious faith with the potential benefits, and it is not useful for the therapist to introduce elements of his or her own philosophy or spiritual system (Cohen 1997; Nelson *et al.* 2002). Therefore, it is important for the therapist to clarify his or her own spiritual outlook, in order to avoid unwittingly imposing it on the therapeutic relationship.

Each medical condition carries with it specific psychosocial implications as well as stressors that are common among broader disease categories. In addition to preparing academically to become familiar with the mechanisms and treatments for the condition that is the focus of one's work, the therapist is advised also to consider his or her own personal history in relation to that illness. Perhaps a family member suffered from, or died from that disease. Perhaps the therapist has risk factors for that condition. These experiences are a source of empathy and effectiveness, as noted above. Unexamined, they can also become a source of disappointment and frustration for the therapist. Motivations, such as repairing the badly handled care of loved ones, or situations where the patient group may come to represent others in the therapist's life, can become an obstacle to effective therapy. We cannot protect our patients from the fear or pain that accompanies living with serious illness. We can, as Deihl put it, learn to be truly present with them, to improve the present and the quality of the time they have for living.

Transference and countertransference issues must be considered in medical DMT, just as in any other application of the modality (Dosamantes-Alperson 1987). There are aspects of the transference dynamic that need special consideration in medical work. For example, Berrol and Katz (1985) raised the provocative and often neglected issue of hate:

> Patients hate the staff for their lack of progress. They believe they are not improving because of the staff's incompetence or willful obstruction. Therapists begin to buy into this hatred. They begin to believe that the patient is not responding to treatment because they are resistant or unmotivated. Therapists feel frustrated and guilty when they imagine that patients are not making progress because of a deficiency in their healing power rather than the nature and extent of the injury... It is important for staff in rehabilitation settings to continually acknowledge that hatred is a normal phenomenon. In this way, the concerns can be openly discussed and feelings dealt with. (Berrol and Katz 1985, p.53)

While the authors of this quotation were discussing the rehabilitation medicine setting, this is relevant to all medical populations. A patient or family member may become jealous of the therapist's health, his or her good fortune in not getting sick. That jealousy can become hostility that will interfere with psychosocial care.

We need to be prepared for this, and as Berrol and Katz advised, accept it as normal without feeling guilty, personalizing the feelings, or internalizing the hatred.

Medical DMT specialists describe the therapeutic relationship as slightly different than in standard psychotherapy contexts. For the most part, therapists relax the role boundaries somewhat. This may take the form of allowing more therapist disclosure. For example, a therapist may attend a funeral and grieve with the family of a deceased patient, or interact in related roles such as at fundraising events (Serlin 1999a). Melsom compared the transference/countertransference dynamic in medical work with that in mental health psychotherapy (1999). She observed that in medical work the therapy is best served if the therapist is more liberal with the transference, and more conservative with his or her own countertransference.

Dance/movement therapists Mowry Rutter (personal communication, July 18, 2002) and Kasovac (personal communication, August 9, 2002) who both work with children, emphasize that the relationship with the ill child's parents is critical. They advise that the therapist needs to be supportive of parents' efforts to manage the multiple stressors in their lives: the child's illness, the needs of other children in the family, their own emotional state, the health of the marriage, their finances and employment. A deep understanding and caring may develop, and at first impression the professional boundaries may look diffuse. However, both specialists caution that, in the best interests of the child, the clinical staff may sometimes need to set a limit or modify a parent's approach. At those times, it is clear that the professional role boundaries must be intact and firm.

Self-care is critical to a therapist's effectiveness and development in this specialty. When patients have life-threatening disease, and sometimes die, their therapists can be left with feelings of helplessness and grief. To fill the gap between what we are able to provide (support, coping strategies, empathy, expression) and what we are not (prolonged life, cure, recovery) some therapists get involved in advocacy work around the disease of concern: a way of bringing balance to work that can be saddening. These activities may include fundraising, speaking engagements or workshops with community advocacy groups, lobbying and so forth. Ongoing exposure to the tragedies of serious illness or injury can bring about compassion fatigue (a combination of burn-out and vicarious traumatization) (Pfifferling and Gilley 2000). Our therapy focuses on the use and experience of the body: our own and our patients'; and in medical work the body is the focus of all other treatment and concern. Theories of somatic countertransference (Dosamantes-Alperson 1987; Pallaro 1994) would suggest that medical dance/movement therapists may be vulnerable to the same feelings of fear, anxiety and defeat that challenge medical patients. To prevent this, therapists and all health care workers can consciously engage in the activities that give life meaning and bring about joy. For dance/movement therapists, this may occur in our own lives as movers and dancers. To combat this, we return to the life-affirming attributes of movement itself. Dance to celebrate the health that you have.

Experiential training exercises

Each of the training exercises presented in this section has been developed to address and illustrate a theoretical construct, an aspect of personal development, or a clinical challenge relevant to medical DMT. For each, a brief introduction relates the learning activity to the body of knowledge. They are all designed for a group training context. Many of these can be easily adapted to use as a structure for clinical intervention with individuals or groups.

Training exercise: Where does it hurt?

People find it a great relief to see their body's plight portrayed in this form. There can be a sense of empathy, and sometimes humor, between the participants. This activity can also be used as an intervention when the patient cannot move, as a form of receptive movement therapy.

- Work in partners, one in the role of therapist and one in the role of patient. In this exercise, the therapist is the mover and the patient works verbally. This is a dialogue.
- *Patient*: describe for your partner, in words, something that is wrong in your body. Identify a body part or zone or system that has been the site of a recent illness or injury, or simply a place that hurts today.
- *Therapist*: listen, and translate the description into movement for your partner. Dance the problem.
- Have a dialogue during this, with the patient "coaching" the therapist until the dance is a true expression of the body's experience. Together, choreograph the healing of the hurt. Dance the problem and the healing for it in sequence. Keep checking in with each other. Give the dance a title.
- Switch roles and make a dance for the other partner. Then discuss the experience together.

Training exercise: Guided imagery of childhood illness

Most adults can remember the experience of a temporary acute childhood illness. This exercise is designed to generate empathy with medically ill people without probing into any of the learner's current body issues. The facilitator should instruct participants to use memories and images of normal childhood illnesses. That way, in case participants have a history of serious childhood illness, they will not be forced to grapple with those more threatening memories. The exercise also shows a procedure for developing bodily sensed memory from imagery into movement expression.

- Find a comfortable position and bring yourself into a relaxed state, eyes closed.

- In your mind, travel back in time to your childhood and let a memory of a normal childhood sickness come to mind. Perhaps having a fever or the chicken pox, getting tonsils or an appendix removed, perhaps a broken arm or a trip to the emergency room.

- Let yourself remember that time: the sensations, the smells and sounds and people around you. Remember what you felt, what you wondered…were you afraid? Let the images from that experience come alive in your memory. How did you get through that experience? Was there any part of it that was fun?

- From these memories, imagine a movement – a short dance or phrase – that captures the essences of that childhood experience. Right where you are, try putting the feeling of that movement in your body, moving in a small way.

- Then bring yourself out of the reverie and your attention to the here and now. Find space to move in and develop your movement idea into a clear phrase or small dance. Show this and share it with other members of the group, and/or write about it in a journal.

Training exercise: Dancing with limitations

This is adapted from a similar exercise taught by James Murphy, MD, ADTR. In it, learners use the creative techniques of DMT to identify movement resources, a process related to coping and problem solving. Next, the expressive movement repertoire becomes a way to explore emotions in a supportive relational context. Also, able-bodied therapists are given a platform to actively experience physical limitations and enhance empathy with patients who are physically confined or debilitated.

- Work in partners. Partner A "limits" the movement capacities of Partner B using any available props or personal belongings. For example, a scarf may blind someone, or bind the ankles together to inhibit walking, or Partner B may be confined to a chair or to the floor. Partner A should be creative, yet ensure safety, in this process.

- Partner A steps back. The partners each take a quiet minute to themselves to take in the situation.

- Partner A returns in the "therapist" role, and Partner B assumes a "patient" role. Together in these roles, explore the remaining movement possibilities: What can be done? Find the options; play with them; improvise. Use movement for your main communication, speaking when needed to clarify, and ensure physical safety for Partner B.

- Next, shift the improvised role play. Using the movement, explore the feelings connected to the limitations. Partner A helps Partner B access, identify and communicate the emotions that emerge from the experience of being limited this way.

- After a few minutes, bring this to a close. Remove the limiting props from Partner B and briefly discuss the experience with each other. Allow Partner B to speak first, and be sure to include feelings and perceptions about the interactive/relational aspects of the role play.

- Switch roles and repeat the process, including the discussion at the end. If you are working as one of many pairs in a large group, the group should come together so the partners can share their experiences. Consider writing on this in a journal as well.

Training exercise: The coping dance

This exercise is easily adapted to clinical work, as described in Chapter 5. The activities exemplify the concept of self-efficacy, as movers discover within themselves ways to cope with stressors. The link between the stressor and the coping strategy is made sequential and seamless as the dance develops. The task includes the important element of activity, so new and personally meaningful behavior patterns are embodied and practiced in the session. Movers may work alone in this task, and should have an opportunity for discussion and sharing afterwards.

- Think about something that is currently happening in your life that is hard and stressful for you. Something difficult to get through. Develop a movement phrase that embodies and expresses this.

- Next, identify something in your life, or in yourself, that helps you get through times like this. Something that might help you with this difficult problem. Explore that idea in movement until you find a movement phrase that embodies it.

- Now do them both: one and then the other. Go back and forth between the two. Notice the transition between them, feel what's happening as you go from one to the other. Embellish that, and find ways to bridge the three together in a seamless sequence: the movement representing the challenge, the transition, and the movement that represents a way to cope with it. Let this become a "mini-dance" and, as you're moving, think of a title for it.

- After the mover(s) bring the movement process to a close, discussion can begin with sharing the titles of the mini-dances. The therapeutic value of this task is in the discovery of the transition phrases, and productive discussion will focus on the mind/body experience that brings the mover from the problem to successful coping.

The exercises below can be included in training sessions, but are designed for clinical work with patients who have pulmonary disease. For child patients, the scripts may need to be shortened and the language simplified.

DMT-based guided imagery for respiratory functioning

Patients with lung disease are guided through the first of these three scripts, and then one of the other two. After people become familiar with both, they should use their preferred imagery set. Flute music provides good accompaniment to this imagery. It is the instrument of the breath. Remembering the potential for bronchoconstriction during deep relaxation states, any relaxation in this exercise should remain at a moderate level (Mrazek and Klinnert 1991). Guide this imagery with a soft yet clear voice, pausing for your own breath, and to mirror vocally the internal spaciousness you are facilitating. Phrases can be repeated, as repetition helps the patient embed the phrase into his or her own mind/body dialogue.

Note that the emphasis is on the experience of breathing. For people with serious pulmonary disease, the therapist may not want to impose specific counts and holds in the breath pattern. Rather, the visualizations are simply for bringing new sensations and images into a breathing process that is often labored, has been subject to medical assessment, and is associated with anxiety and illness.

The first of the three imagery sets is designed to reflect the physiological process of breathing and aims at anatomical correctness. The second emphasizes the continuity and ease of breathing while suggesting subtle postural adjustments to support the breath function. The third draws upon the concept of three-dimensionality in space and in body shaping (Amighi *et al.* 1999; Kestenberg 1975). Each of these sequences should be preceded by a brief induction for calming, centering and grounding the body and bringing the mind's focus to the breath. Each can be concluded with either a gentle return to normal awareness, or developed into movement that would amplify and externalize the internal, imagined movement themes.

OPENING THE ALVEOLI

Begin to watch the pathway of the breath. Bring in the air through the mouth or nose. See the airways in your mind's eye. Follow the breath in and down. Where the airways branch out and get smaller, let the air flow into each branch, and all the way into the lungs. See your lungs as sponges, with lots of little spaces. The spaces are filling with breath. See the air enter and open those spaces to do its good work, and leave again fully, all the way out of the body. Imagine the spaces down in your lungs growing larger, receiving more air, each time a little bit more. If there's a place that feels tight, concentrate your attention there, and watch the spaces open to the breath. See that part of your lung become more receptive, and loosening.

Let the breaths easily flow upwards and out, traveling through the pathways as they converge and widen, and through your mouth or nose. Breath traveling downwards and in, upwards and out. For a few minutes, just follow the pathway of your own breath at your own pace.

THE BICYCLE CHAIN

Bring your attention to the transitions in your breathing, the transition between inhaling and exhaling. Allow the transitions to be rounded and smooth, rather than jagged and cornered. Let the inhale simply become the exhale, let the exhale become the inhale. Ride that transition in a smooth and rounded way…almost like a circle of breath. So you breathe a round breath. In your mind's eye, see the circle of breath moving up the front of your torso, and down the back, with smooth rounded transitions. Up the front, curving over the shoulders and down the back, curving up and forward at the bottom and around again...like a bicycle chain. Take a few breaths in your own pace, and follow the breath around on that pathway... See the bicycle chain and then, in your mind's eye, put one twist in the chain...it is now a figure 8 in the middle of the torso. Let the breath ride the curving, looping pathways of the figure 8...watch the breath as it does that. Let the image of the figure 8 float around inside your middle body space, taking the breath into all the places it can go... Bring the image back to the center, let the chain open into a single circular loop again...rounded, smooth transitions...and find a breath rhythm that is comfortable for you.

3D BREATHING

With your inhaling, imagine that you are filling more and more of your torso with air. Imagine the air filling all the way down to the base of your body, into your back, into your belly. Visualize the middle body as one big open space, able to use the air. Imagine the length of that inner space like a cylinder, and with a very slight movement of your spine, lengthen upwards as you inhale...condense and come downward as you exhale, shortening a little. So each time you inhale and exhale, you're moving upwards and downwards with your spine...feel that change in your body shape support the breath.

Then imagine the width of your body from side to side. See the space inside your rib cage, the spaces between each pair of ribs, the width around your waist...as you inhale, fill sideways and widen. See if you can stretch a little out to your sides – both directions at the same time. When you exhale, narrow and close around the center, as though your ribs were going to meet and knit together. Focus your breathing sideways, widening and narrowing with a very slight movement, feeling your width and the center of your breath.

Now feel the depth of your body...the space between your belly button and your backbone. And as you breath in, fill forwards...exhale and hollow backwards and feel concave. Support your breath by growing forwards and filling when you inhale and small movements backwards to empty when you exhale... Then imagine all three dimensions of space inside...lengthening, filling sideways and forwards when you inhale, and when you exhale condensing down, narrowing and hollowing. The muscles in your torso respond and change with each breath.

Multidisciplinarity revisited

The medical DMT specialists interviewed for this text asserted the importance of a multidisciplinary perspective. Specifically, one must keep in mind the fact that, in this application, the medical priorities are the clinical priorities. Patients are there for a restoration of physical health. As psychosocial service providers we are there because our services are but one of many means to that end. Theoretically, this may mean adjusting treatment goals more toward coping, comfort and support, as described in earlier chapters. On a practical level, this often means adjusting one's clinical work to the irregular and sometimes impromptu scheduling of activities on a medical unit.

The medical system, like any system, is hierarchical in nature. It behooves the therapist working in the field to learn about the roles of other professionals and how clinical work is distributed among different professional groups in the particular setting. For example, nurse practitioners and physician assistants may have very similar roles or quite diverse responsibilities depending on the facility. Nurses are by no means a homogenous professional group in health care and may be educated to certificate level, bachelor's degree, Master's or doctoral-level education, with levels of responsibility spanning the entire hierarchy. Some hospitals are equipped with both health psychology and social work departments, and psychosocial care is distributed between these groups. DMT may be housed with either, or in pediatric settings with a Child Life department.

Mastering the ins and outs of a medical infrastructure is one aspect of integrating DMT into the health care program. It is even more important to develop collaborative, collegial relationships that best serve the needs of patients and their families. Using the knowledge acquired in formal learning will support those relationships. The creative arts therapist may initially feel out of place in the medical setting, and may need to persist with constructing and clarifying a professional role (Keenan 1997). Schwartz (1982) envisioned the biopsychosocial health care team this way:

> If a given specialist has not been formally trained biopsychosocially in terms of content and clinical skills...then this health provider should be content to be "part" of the "whole", and not attempt to represent the "whole" in terms of practice and responsibility... The well-rounded physician of the future, trained in the interdisciplinary profession of medicine rather than in the discipline of biology, psychology, or sociology per se, becomes the person best equipped to take legal and ethical responsibility for integrating and coordinating the patient's care biopsychosocially. (Schwartz 1982, p.1051)

This view places the physician at the top of the health care team, but acknowledges the need for all team members to adopt the biopsychosocial approach. Employing Engel's systems hierarchy (see Chapter 4), Schwartz advises that each member of the team receive training above and below one's level of practice (1982, p.1045). Dance/movement therapists generally intervene at the level of the person, the two-person dyad or the family. Thus, our training for medical work should include information at the nervous and (if possible) organ system levels, as well as at the community and (if possible) culture/subculture levels.

Jemmott stated, "No one profession can be totally responsible for a patient's care. Each profession contributes its expertise" (Jemmott 1985, p.505). This text has attempted to describe the expertise that DMT brings to general medical care, and how it might best be contributed.

Additional Resources for Medical Dance/Movement Therapists

American Psychological Association
Division 38, Health Psychology
American Psychological Association
750 First Street, NE
Washington, District of Columbia 20002-4242
Phone: (202) 336-6013
www.apa.org/about/div38
www.health-psych.org

American Psychosomatic Society
6728 Old McLean Village Drive
McLean, Virginia 22101-3906
Phone: (703) 556-9222
www.psychosomatic.org

The American Psychosomatic Society is a forum for the discussion of data, from any discipline, that may enhance our understanding of the complex relationships which have led to a new appreciation of how mind and body interact in the maintenance of health and the causation of disease.

Association for Dance Movement Therapy, UK
www.admt.org.uk

Australian Dance Therapy Association
www.dtaa.org

Brecha – Dance Movement Therapy en Argentina
www.brecha.com.ar

Cochrane Collaboration Complementary Medicine
Dr. Brian Berman
Complementary Field Co-ordinator
University of Maryland School of Medicine
Kernan Hospital Mansion
3rd Floor
2200 N Forest Park Avenue
Baltimore, Maryland

Phone: (410) 448-6871
Fax: (410) 448-6875
www.cochrane.org

The Cochrane Collaboration is an international research group that produces and disseminates systematic reviews of health care interventions and promotes the search for evidence in the form of clinical trials and other studies of interventions, including complementary therapies.

German Dance Therapy Association
Feldstr. 35
21335 Lueneburg
Germany
Phone: 04131/78 92 96
Fax: 04131/78 92 96
www.dancetherapy.de

International Psycho-Oncology Society (IPOS)
www.ipos-society.org

Founded in 1984, IPOS is the international colleague organization of the American Psycho-Oncology Society. Membership is open to individuals with a diversity of clinical an research backgrounds and offers them the opportunity to network with professionals in their fields from around the world.

Japan Dance Therapy Association
www.jadta.net/dance/jadta_english.html

National Center for Complementary and Alternative Medicine
National Institutes of Health
Bethesda, Maryland 20892
www.nccam.nih.gov

Society for the Arts and Healthcare Japan
Email: art-care@popo.or.jp

Society for the Arts in Healthcare
1632 U Street, NW
Washington, District of Columbia 20009
Phone: (202) 244-8088
www.theSAH.org

The SAH is "dedicated to promoting the incorporation of the arts as an appropriate and integral component of healthcare."

The Society of Behavioral Medicine
7600 Terrace Ave, Suite 203
Middleton, Wisconsin 53562
Phone: (608) 827-7267
www.sbm.org

SBM is a "scientific forum for over 3000 behavioral and biomedical researchers and clinicians to study the interactions of behavior, physiological and biochemical states, and morbidity and mortality".

Biographies of Foreword Writer and Medical Dance/Movement Therapy Interviewees

John Graham-Pole MBBS MRCP MD graduated from St Bartholomew's Hospital, University of London, in October 1966. He became a member of the Royal College of Physicians in 1970, and board certified in Child Health and Pediatrics in both Britain and America. He defended his dissertation in medicine at London University in 1978. He has been on the faculty of three universities since 1976, specializing in Pediatric Hematology and Oncology.

He is professor of Pediatrics and affiliate professor of Clinical and Health Psychology at the University of Florida in Gainesville. He co-founded Shands Hospital Arts in Medicine in 1991and is its medical director. He is co-director of the university's Center for the Arts & Health Research and Education, and on the advisory boards of the university's Center for Spirituality and Health and the National Society for the Arts in Healthcare. He directs the Children's Hospice of North Central Florida and the Shands Children's Hospital Palliative Care Consultation Service.

Judith Richardson Bunney MA ADTR served as Director of Dance/Movement Therapy at the District of Columbia Department of Mental Health Services, which includes St. Elizabeths Hospital, considered to be the birthplace of modern dance/movement therapy. She has a private practice working with creative blocks, giving grief workshops, and has expertise as a trainer in team building and group dynamics. She specializes in treating forensic and geropsychiatric clients. A professional DMT for over 45 years, a founding member and Past President of the American Dance Therapy Association, she has taught in several European DMT programs.

Linni Deihl MEd ADTR has worked as a dance/movement therapist since 1964. For 27 years she has taught an intensive summer course in DMT, and also in several university settings. She maintains a private practice specializing in psychogenic somatic disorders, and works in hospice care with cardiac, cancer and AIDS patients. She also works as a choreographer and dance educator.

Susan Imus ADTR GLCMA LCP is currently the Chairperson of the Dance/Movement Therapy Department in the Graduate School at Columbia College Chicago. Susan was one of the founders of the Harvard Community Health Plan's Pain Program in Boston, and Clinical Manager from 1988–94. Her medical DMT background also includes work at the New England Rehabilitation Hospital and Northwest Community Hospital in Des Moines, Iowa. She holds a graduate certificate in art therapy.

Nicholas G. Kasovac MA DTR CMT LMT provided DMT and massage therapy services to the Pediatric Pain Program at UCLA Children's Hospital in outpatient, inpatient and intensive care settings. He is also certified in therapeutic touch. He is currently with the Outpatient Desert Samaritan Medical Center in Mesa, Arizona in the Outpatient Pediatric Pain Center.

Patricia Mowry Rutter MA CMA ADTR LPC served as dance/movement therapist for the Pediatric Day Program at the National Jewish Medical Center in Denver, Colorado, where she worked with children from the ages of one month to twenty years. Also trained in yoga and Authentic Movement, she is currently teaching and consulting in the Denver area.

References

Achterberg, J. (1985) *Imagery in Healing: Shamanism and Modern Medicine*. Boston, MA: Shambhala.

Achterberg, J., Dossey, L., Gordon, J. S., Hegedus, C., Herrman, M. W. and Nelson, R. (1994) "Mind–body interventions." In B. M. Berman and D. B. Larson (eds) *Alternative Medicine: Expanding Medical Horizons: A Report to the NIH on Alternative Medical Systems and Practices in the US, Prepared under the Auspices of the Workshop on Alternative Medicine*. Washington, DC: U.S. Government Printing Office, National Institutes of Health.

Achterberg, J. and Lawlis, G. F. (1978) *Imagery of Cancer: Image–CA: An Evaluation Tool for the Process of Disease*. Champaign, IL: Institute for Personality and Ability Testing.

Adams, P. and Mylander, M. (1993) *Gesundheit!* Rochester, VT: Healing Arts Press.

Ader, R. (1996) "Historical perspectives on psychoneuroimmunology." In H. Friedman, T. W. Klein and A. L. Friedman (eds) *Psychoneuroimmunology, Stress and Infection*. Boca Raton, FL: CRC Press.

Aldridge, D. (1994) "Single-case research design for the creative art therapist." *The Arts in Psychotherapy: An International Journal, 21*, 5, 333–42.

American Dance Therapy Association (ADTA) (2002) "What is dance/movement Therapy?" Retrieved July 17, 2002, from the World Wide Web: www.adta.org

American Psychiatric Association (APA) (1994) *Diagnostic and Statistical Manual of Mental Disorders* (4th ed.). Washington, DC: American Psychiatric Association.

American Psychological Association (APA) (n.d.) "American Psychological Association (APA), Division 38, Health Psychology." Retrieved July 18, 2002, from the World Wide Web: www.apa.org

Amighi, J. K., Loman, S., Lewis, P. and Sossin, K. M. (1999) *The Meaning of Movement: Developmental and Clinical Perspectives of the Kestenberg Movement Profile*. Amsterdam: Gordon and Breach Publishers.

Ascheim, F., Meizel Binder, M., Coolidge, L. and Leavitt, J. (1992) "At the growing edge of dance/movement therapy: Working in the rehabilitation setting." Paper presented at the American Dance Therapy Association 27th Annual Conference, October, Columbia, MD.

Asthma and Allergy Foundation of America (2002) "Asthma and allergies: Asthma facts." Retrieved September 1, 2002, from the World Wide Web: www.aafa.org

Baider, L., Peretz, T., Hadani, P. E. and Koch, U. (2001) "Psychological intervention in cancer patients: a randomized study." *General Hospital Psychiatry, 23*, 272–7.

Bandler, R., and Grindler, J. (1979). *Frogs into Princes: Neuro Linguistic Programming*. Moab, Utah: Real People Press.

Barker, L. R., Burton, J. R. and Zieve, P. D. (eds) (1982) *Principles of Ambulatory Medicine*. Baltimore, MD: Williams and Wilkins.

Barlow, L. C. (1983) "Effects of dance/movement therapy on fear in asthmatic children." Unpublished Master's thesis, Antioch New England Graduate School, Keene, NH. Abstracted in A.C. Fisher and A. Stark (eds) (1998) *Dance/Movement Therapy Abstracts: Doctoral Dissertations, Masters' Theses, and Special Projects, Volume 1.* Columbia, MD: Marian Chace Foundation, ADTA.

Barsky, A. and Baszender, I. (1998) "Perspectives on pain-related suffering: Presentations and discussions." *Advances in Mind–Body Medicine, 14* (Summer), 167–203.

Bartenieff, I. (1974) "Space, effort and the brain." *Main Currents in Modern Thought, 31,* 1, 36–9.

Bartenieff, I. (with Lewis, Dori) (1980) *Body movement: Coping with the Environment.* New York: Gordon and Breach Science Publishers.

Basmajian, J. V. and Blumenstein, R. (1980) *Electrode placement in EMG Biofeedback.* Baltimore, MD: Williams & Wilkins.

Battino, R. (2001) *Guided Imagery and Other Approaches to Healing.* Bancyfelin, UK: Crown House Publishing.

Baum, A. (1990) "Stress, intrusive imagery, and chronic distress." *Health Psychology, 9,* 6, 653–75.

Belar, C. D. and Geisser, M. E. (1995) "Roles of the clinical health psychologist in the management of chronic illness." In P. M. Nicassio and T. W. Smith (eds) *Managing Chronic Illness: A Biopsychosocial Perspective.* Washington, DC: American Psychological Association.

Belsky, J. and Khanna, P. (1994) "The effects of self-hypnosis for children with cystic fibrosis: A pilot study." *American Journal of Clinical Hypnosis, 36,* 282–92

Benioff, L. R. and Vinogradov, S. (1993) "Group psychotherapy with cancer patients and the terminally ill." In H. I. Kaplan and B. J. Sadock (eds) *Comprehensive Group Psychotherapy* (3rd ed.). Baltimore, MD: Williams and Wilkins.

Benjamin, H. H. (1987) *From Victim to Victor: The Wellness Community Guide to Fighting for Recovery for Cancer Patients and their Families.* New York: Dell Publishing.

Benson, H. (1975) *The Relaxation Response.* New York: Avon Books.

Berkman, L. (1995) "The role of social relations in health promotion." *Psychosomatic Medicine, 57,* 245–54.

Bernstein, P. L. (1980) "A mythologic quest: Jungian movement therapy with the pyschosomatic client." *American Journal of Dance Therapy, 3,* 2, 44–55.

Bernstein, P. L. and Cafarelli, E. (1972) "An electromyographical validation of the effort system of notation." *Writings on Body Movement and Communication,* ADTA Monograph No. 2, 78–94.

Berrol, C. F. (1992) "The neurophysiologic basis of the mind–body connection in dance/movement therapy." *American Journal of Dance Therapy, 14,* 1, 19–29.

Berrol, C. F. (2000) "The spectrum of research options in dance/movement therapy." *American Journal of Dance Therapy, 22,* 1, 29–46.

Berrol, C. F. and Katz, S. S. (1985) "Dance/movement therapy in the rehabilitation of individuals surviving severe head injuries." *American Journal of Dance Therapy, 8,* 46–66.

Berrol, C. F., Katz, S. S., Lombardo, N. E. and Ooi, W. L. (1996) *Dance/Movement Therapy with Older Individuals who have Sustained Neurological Insult,* Final Report, Administration on Aging Grant Number 90 AM 0669, Columbia, MD: American Dance Therapy Association.

Berrol, C. F., Ooi, W. L. and Katz, S. S. (1997) "Dance/movement therapy with older adults who have sustained neurological insult: A demonstration project." *American Journal of Dance Therapy, 19,* 2, 135–60.

Berry, D. S. and Pennebaker, J. W. (1993) "Nonverbal and verbal emotional expression and health." *Psychotherapy and Psychosomatics, 59*, 11–19.

von Bertalanffy, L. (1968) *General Systems Theory.* New York: Braziller.

Bibace, R. and Walsh, M. E. (1978) "Developmental stages in children's conceptions of illness." In G. Stone, F. Cohen and N. Adler (eds) *Health Psychology: A Handbook.* San Francisco, CA: Jossey-Bass.

Bibace, R. and Walsh, M. E. (1980) "Development of children's concept of illness." *Pediatrics, 66*, 912–17.

Billings, D. W., Folkman, S., Acree, M. and Moskowitz, J. T. (2000) "Coping and physical health during caregiving: The roles of positive and negative affect" [electronic version]. *Journal of Personality and Social Psychology, 79*, 1, 131–42.

Birdwhistell, R. (1970) *Kinesics and Context.* Philadelphia, PA: University of Pennsylvania Press.

Bittman, B. B., Berk, L. S., Felten, D. L., Westengard, J., Simonton, O. C., Pappas, J. and Ninehouser, M. (2001) "Composite effects of group drumming music therapy on modulation of neuroendocrine-immune parameters in normal subjects." *Alternative Therapies in Health and Medicine, 7*, 1, 38–47.

Blaney, P. H. (1985) "Psychological considerations in cancer." In N. Schneiderman and J. Tapp (eds) *Behavioral Medicine: The Biopsychosocial Approach.* Hillsdale, NJ: Lawrence Erlbaum Associates Publishers.

Blau, B. and Siegel, E. V. (1978) "Breathing together: A preliminary investigation of an involuntary reflex as adaptation." *American Journal of Dance Therapy, 2*, 1, 35–42.

Blumenthal, S. J., Matthews, K. and Weiss, S. M. (eds) (1993) *New Research Frontiers in Behavioral Medicine: Proceedings of the National Conference.* Chantilly, VA: U.S. Government Printing Office, NIH/NIMH.

Bojner-Horwitz, E., Theorell, T. and Anderberg, U. M. (2003) "Dance/movement therapy and changes in stress-related hormones: A study of fibromyalgia patients with video-interpretation." *The Arts in Psychotherapy: An International Journal, 30*, 5, 255–64.

Bovbjerg, D. H. and Stone, A. A. (1996) "Psychological stress and upper respiratory illness." In H. Friedman, T. W. Klein and A. L. Friedman (eds) *Psychoneuroimmunology, Stress and Infection.* Boca Raton, FL: CRC Press.

Bowers, M. R., Swan, J. E. and Koehler, W. F. (1994) "What attributes determine quality and satisfaction with health care delivery?" [electronic version]. *Health Care Management Review, 19*, 4, 49–55.

Brauninger, I. (2000) "Stress management and improvement of quality of life through dance therapy: A controlled empirical study." Research poster presented at the American Dance Therapy Association 35th Annual Conference, October, Seattle, WA.

Brody, D. (1998) "Mental health issues in the primary care setting." Paper presented at the Mind/Body Symposium Series, MCP Hahnemann University, March, Philadelphia, PA.

Bronfenbrenner, U. (1979) *The Ecology of Human Development: Experiments by Nature and Design.* Cambridge, MA: Harvard University Press.

Brooks, D. and Stark, A. (1989) "The effect of D/MT on affect: A pilot study." *American Journal of Dance Therapy, 11*, 2, 101–11.

Bunney, J. R. (2000) "Dealing with loss through body movement and dance." Paper presented at the American Dance Therapy Association 35th Annual Conference, October, Seattle, WA.

Burn, H. (1987) "The movement behavior of anorectics: The control issue." *American Journal of Dance Therapy, 10,* 54–76.

Burns, C. (1996) "Comparative analysis of humor versus relaxation training for the enhancement of immunocompetence (immune deficiency)." Unpublished doctoral dissertation, Biola University.

Burns, S. J. I., Harbuz, M. S., Hucklebridge, F. and Bunt, L. (2001) "A pilot study into the therapeutic effects of music therapy at a cancer help center." *Alternative Therapies in Health and Medicine, 7,* 1, 48–56.

Caldwell, C. (2001) "The biology of creative states." Paper presented at the American Dance Therapy Association 36th Annual Conference, October, Raleigh, NC.

Cannon, L., Hammond, M., Kasovac, N., Meizel Binder, M., Petrone, K. and Pratson, D. (1997) "Dance/movement therapy as a psychosocial service in medical settings." Paper presented at the American Dance Therapy Association 32nd Annual Conference, November, Philadelphia, PA.

Cannon, W. B. (1932) *The Wisdom of the Body.* New York: W.W. Norton and Co., Inc.

Carver, C., Scheier, M. and Weintraub, J. K. (1989) "Assessing coping strategies: A theoretically based approach." *Journal of Personality and Social Psychology, 56,* 2, 267–83.

Cash, T. F. and Pruzinsky, T. (eds) (1990) *Body Images: Development, Deviance and Change.* New York: The Guilford Press.

Cassidy, C. M., Cassileth, B., Jonas, W., Pavek, R. and Silversmith, L. (1994) "A guide for the alternative researcher." In B. M. Berman and D. B. Larson (eds) *Alternative Medicine: Expanding Medical Horizons: A Report to the NIH on Alternative Medical Systems and Practices in the U.S.* Washington, DC: U.S. Government Printing Office, National Institutes of Health.

Cassileth, B., Jonas, W. and Cassidy, C. M. (1994) "Research methodologies." In B. M. Berman and D. B. Larson (eds) *Alternative Medicine: Expanding Medical Horizons: A Report to the NIH on Alternative Medical Systems and Practices in the U.S.* Washington, DC: U.S. Government Printing Office, National Institutes of Health.

Center for Mind/Body Medicine, Harvard University Medical Center (1999) "About Mind/Body Medicine." Retrieved October 11, 1999, from the World Wide Web: www.mbmi.org

Chaiklin, H. (1994) "The crossroads of dance therapy." *American Journal of Dance Therapy, 16,* 2, 71–80.

Chaiklin, H. (2000) "Doing case study research." *American Journal of Dance Therapy, 22,* 1, 47–59.

Chaiklin, S. and Schmais, C. (1993) "The Chace approach to dance therapy." In S. Sandel, S. Chaiklin and A. Lohn (eds) *Foundations of Dance/Movement Therapy: The Life and Work of Marian Chace.* Columbia, MD: American Dance Therapy Association.

Chang, M. (1997) "Dance/movement therapy + Mindfulness Meditation = Mindful Moving." Paper presented at the American Dance Therapy Association 32nd Annual Conference, November, Philadelphia, PA.

Chatfield, S. J. (1998) "Neuromuscular patterns in movement: Moments of choice or habit?" Paper presented at the Congress on Research in Dance Annual Conference, Ohio State University.

Chodorow, J. (1995) "Body, psyche, and the emotions." *American Journal of Dance Therapy, 17,* 2, 97–114.

Chopra, D. (n.d.) "About mind/body medicine." Retrieved October 11, 1999, from the World Wide Web: www.chopra.com

Coburn, L. (1995) "Experiencing and transforming: Dance therapy imagery of an HIV+ client." Unpublished Master's thesis, Hunter College, CUNY, New York. Abstracted in Fisher and Stark (eds) (1998) *Dance/Movement Therapy Abstracts: Doctoral Dissertations, Masters' Theses, and Special Projects, Volume 2*. Columbia, MD: Marian Chace Foundation, ADTA.

Cohen, R. (1991) "The effects of psychological intervention (using guided imagery) on responses to ragweed-pollen nasal challenge in allergic subjects." Unpublished doctoral dissertation, The Union Institute, Cincinnati, OH.

Cohen, S. (1988) "Psychosocial models of the role of social support in the etiology of physical disease." *Health Psychology, 7*, 3, 269–97.

Cohen, S. O. (1996) "Before the stillness: Dance therapy helps the young communicate before they die." *Hospice, 5*.

Cohen, S. O. (1997) "Spirituality and healing." *The Research Connection: Newsletter of the Psychosocial Nursing Advisory Group to the New Jersey State Commission on Cancer Research, 3*, 1–4.

Cohen, S. O. and Walco, G. A. (1999) "Dance/movement therapy for children and adolescents with cancer." *Cancer Practice, 7*, 1, 34–42.

Coleman, J. M., Pratt, R. R., Stoddard, R.A., Gerstmann, D.R. and Abel, H.H. (1998) "The effects of the male and female singing and speaking voices on selected physiological and behavioral measures of premature infants in the intensive care unit." *International Journal of Arts Medicine, 5*, 2, 4–11.

Comer, M. E. (1992) "Dance therapy and gay men with AIDS". Unpublished Master's thesis, Hunter College, CUNY, New York. Abstracted in Fisher and Stark (eds) (1998) *Dance/Movement Therapy Abstracts: Doctoral Dissertations, Masters' Theses, and Special Projects, Volume 2*. Columbia, MD: Marian Chace Foundation, ADTA.

Condon, W. S. (1968) *Linguistic-Kinesic Research and dance therapy. ADTA Monograph No. 3*, 21–42.

Condon, W. S. and Ogston, W. D. (1969) "Speech and body motion synchrony of the speaker-hearer." In P. Kjeldergaard (ed.) *Perception of Language*. Columbus, OH: Merrill Books.

Cotman, C. W., Brinton, R. E., Galaburda, A., McEwen, B. and Schneider, D. M. (1987) *The Neuro-Immune-Endocrine Connection*. New York: Raven Press.

Coyne, J. (2000) "Social relationships, distress, and survival among CHF patients." Paper presented at the Mind/Body Programs Symposium Series, February, MCP Hahnemann University, Philadelphia, PA.

Cresswell, J. W. (1998) *Qualitative Inquiry and Research Design: Choosing Among Five Traditions*. Thousand Oaks, CA: Sage Publications, Inc.

Cruz, R. and Sabers, D. (1998) "Dance/movement therapy is more effective than previously reported." *The Arts in Psychotherapy: An International Journal, 25*, 101–104.

Csikszentmihalyi, M. (1990) *Flow: The Psychology of Optimal Experience*. New York: Harper and Row, Inc.

Darby, B. R. (1990) "The effects of psychological intervention on the immune response." Unpublished doctoral dissertation, University of Florida, Gainesville, FL.

Davis, M. (1990) "Laban Movement Analysis and behavioral research: Metatheory implications." In M. Eddy (ed.) *LMA Compendium*. New York: Laban/Bartenieff Institute of Movement Studies.

Davis, M. (1991) "Guide to movement analysis methods." Unpublished manuscript, available from the author. New York.

Davis, M. and Hadiks, D. (1990) "Nonverbal behavior and client state change during psychotherapy." *Journal of Clinical Psychology, 46,* 340–51.

Davis, M. and Hadiks, D. (1994) "Nonverbal aspects of therapist attunement." *Journal of Clinical Psychology, 50,* 3, 393–405.

Davis, S. L. (2002) *Thriving after Breast Cancer: Essential Healing Exercises for Body and Mind.* New York: Broadway Books.

Dayanim, S. (1998) "Image stories: Towards the movement assessment of effort production." Unpublished Master's thesis, MCP Hahnemann University, Philadelphia, PA.

Dell, C. (1970) *A Primer for Movement Description: Using Effort/Shape and Supplementary Concepts.* New York: Dance Notation Bureau.

Detmar, S. B., Muller, M. J., Wever, L. D., Schornagel, J. H. and Aaronson, N. K. (2001) "Patient–physician communication during outpatient palliative treatment visits." *Journal of the American Medical Association, 285,* 10, 1351–7.

Dibbel-Hope, S. (2000) "The use of dance/movement therapy in psychological adaptation to breast cancer." *The Arts in Psychotherapy: An International Journal, 27,* 1, 51–68.

Deihl, L. (1992) "The dying process humanized through body empathy." Paper presented at the American Dance Therapy Association 27th Annual Conference, October, Columbia, MD.

Dienstfrey, H. E. (2001) "An Advances Forum: The state of the science: The best evidence for the involvement of thoughts and feelings in physical health" [feature article]. *Advances in Mind–Body Medicine, 17,* 2–59.

Dieterich, H. (1990) "The art of healing: A mulitmodal treatment approach to cancer using dance/movement therapy and imagery." Unpublished Master's thesis, California State University Hayward, Hayward, CA.

Dijkwel, J. J. (1998) "The Functional Assessment of Movement and Perception (FAMP) as an indicator of change: A multiple case study using a model of brief DMT with traumatic and acquired brain injured adults." Unpublished Master's thesis, MCP Hahnemann University, Philadelphia, PA.

DiMatteo, M. R. (1995) "Health psychology research: The interpersonal challenges." In G. G. Brannigan and M. R. Merrens (eds) *The Social Psychologists: Research Adventures.* New York: McGraw-Hill Book Company.

DiMatteo, M. R., Hays, R. D. and Prince, L. M. (1986) "Relationship of physician's nonverbal communication skill to patient satisfaction, appointment noncompliance, and physician workload." *Health Psychology, 5,* 6, 581–94.

Dosamantes, I. (1992) "Body image: Repository for cultural idealizations and denigrations of the self." *The Arts in Psychotherapy: An International Journal, 19,* 257–67.

Dosamantes-Alperson, E. (1987) "Transference and countertransference issues in movement psychotherapy." *The Arts in Psychotherapy: An International Journal, 14,* 209–14.

Dossey, L. (2001) "Creativity: On intelligence, insight and the cosmic soup." *Choices, 1,* 1, 5–6.

Dulicai, B. D. (1995) "Movement indicators of attention and their role as identifiers of lead exposure." Unpublished doctoral dissertation, The Union Institute, Cincinnati, OH.

Dulicai, D. (1977) "Nonverbal assessment of family systems: Clinical implications." *The Arts in Psychotherapy: An International Journal, 6,* 55–62.

Dunn, A. J. (1996) "Psychoneuroimmunology, stress and infection." In H. Friedman, T. W. Klein and A. L. Friedman (eds) *Psychoneuroimmunology, Stress and Infection.* Boca Raton, FL: CRC Press.

Edwards, A. (2000) "2000 years of treating pain." *Analgesia, 11,* 1, 8–13.

Eisenberg, D.M., Kessler, R.C., Foster, C., Norlock, F.E., Calkins, D.R., and Delbanco, T.L. (1993) "Unconventional Medicine in the United States: Prevalence, Costs and Patterns of Use." *New England Journal of Medicine, 328,* 4, 246–252.

Engel, G. L. (1977) "The need for a new medical model: A challenge for biomedicine." *Science, 196,* 4286, 129–36.

Engel, G. L. (1980) "The clinical application of the biopsychosocial model." *American Journal of Psychiatry, 137,* 5, 535–44.

Erwin-Grabner, T., Goodill, S., Schelly Hill, E. and VonNeida, K. (1999) "Effectiveness of dance/movement therapy on reducing test anxiety." *American Journal of Dance Therapy, 21,* 1, 19–34.

Esterling, B. A. (1991) "Relaxation and exercise intervention as a means of modulating antibody to Epstein-Barr and Human Herpes Virus Type-6 in an asymptomative HIV-1 seropositive and seronegative cohort." Unpublished doctoral dissertation, University of Miami, Miami, FL.

Farber, N. J. (2002) "Giving support when giving the diagnosis of cancer." *Delaware Medical Journal, 74,* 4, 187–9.

Farber, N. J., Novack, D. H. and O'Brien, M. K. (1997) "Love, boundaries and the patient–physician relationship." *Archives of Internal Medicine, 157,* 2291–4.

Fawzy, F. I. and Fawzy, N. W. (1994) "Psychoeducational interventions and health outcomes." In R. Glaser and J. M. Kiecolt-Glaser (eds) *Handbook of Human Stress and Immunity.* San Diego, CA: Academic Press.

Fehder, W. P. and Douglas, S. D. (2001) "Interactions between the nervous and immune systems." *Seminars in Clinical Neuropsychiatry, 6,* 4, 229–40.

Field, T., Morrow, C., Valdeon, C., Larson, S., Kuhn, C. and Schanberg, S. (1992) "Massage reduces anxiety in child and adolescent psychiatry patients." *Journal of the American Academy of Child Adolescent Psychiatry, 31,* 125–31.

Field, T., Quintino, O., Henteleff, T., Wells-Keife, L. and Delvecchio-Feinberg, G. (1997) "Job stress reduction techniques." *Alternative Therapies in Health and Medicine, 3,* 4, 54–6.

Field, T. M., Martinez, A., Nawrocki, T., Pickens, J., Fox, N. A. and Schanberg, S. (1998) "Music shifts frontal EEG in depressed adolescents." *Adolescence, 33,* 129, 109–16.

Finisdore, E. A. (1997) "A comparison of authentic movement with authentic movement under a hypnotic trance." Unpublished Master's thesis, Allegheny University of the Health Sciences, Philadelphia, PA.

Fisher, S. and Cleveland, S. E. (1968) *Body Image and Personality* (2nd ed.). New York: Dover Publications.

Fitzgerald, J. (2000) "Dance/movement therapy and a psychoeducational curriculum on death, dying, and loss: Effects of cognitive and emotional understanding for adults with mental retardation." Research poster session abstracts from the 1999 and 2000 conferences. *American Journal of Dance Therapy, 22,* 2, 132.

Foglietti, R. (1995) "Dance/movement therapy and hope in people living with AIDS." Unpublished Master's thesis, Naropa Institute, Boulder, CO. Abstracted in Fisher and Stark (eds) (1998) *Dance/Movement Therapy Abstracts: Doctoral Dissertations, Masters' Theses, and Special Projects, Volume 2.* Columbia, MD: Marian Chace Foundation, ADTA.

Folkman, S. and Moskowitz, J. T. (2000) "Positive affect and the other side of coping." *American Psychologist, 55*, 6, 647–54.

Fraenkel, D. (1983) "The relationship of empathy in movement to synchrony, echoing, and empathy in verbal interactions." *American Journal of Dance Therapy, 6,* 31–48.

Fraenkel, D. L. (1986) "The ins and outs of medical encounters: An interactional analysis of empathy, patient satisfaction, and information exchange." Unpublished doctoral dissertation, University of Rochester, Rochester, NY.

Frankenhaeuser, M. (1983) "The sympathetic-adrenal and pituitary-adrenal response to challenge: Comparison between the sexes." In M. Dembroski, T. H. Schmidt and G. Blumchen (eds) *Biobehavioral Bases of Coronary Heart Disease.* Basel: Karger.

Franklin, S. (1979) "Movement therapy and selected measures of body image in the trainable mentally retarded." *American Journal of Dance Therapy, 3,* 1, 43–50.

Freeman, L. W. and Lawlis, G. F. (2001) *Mosby's Complementary and Alternative Medicine: A Research-based Approach.* St. Louis, MO: Mosby.

Freud, A. (1979) *Ego and Mechanisms of Defense* (Vol. 2). New York: International Universities Press (original work published 1936).

Friedman, H., Klein, T. W. and Friedman, A. L. (1996) *Psychoneuroimmunology, Stress and Infection.* Boca Raton, FL: CRC Press.

Friedman, R., Myers, P., Krass, S. and Benson, H. (1996) "The relaxation response: Use with cardiac patients." In R. Allen and S. S. Scheidt (eds) *Heart and Mind: The Practice of Cardiac Psychology.* Washington, DC: American Psychological Association.

Friedman, R., Sobel, D. S., Myers, P., Caudill, M. and Benson, H. (1995) "Behavioral medicine, clinical health psychology, and cost offset." *Health Psychology, 14,* 6, 509–18.

Furniss, C. K. (1998) "The use of the expressive arts therapies in chronic pain management and treatment." Unpublished Master's thesis, California State University, Long Beach, CA.

Futterman, A. D., Kemeny, M. E., Shapiro, D., Polonsky, W. and Fahey, J. (1992) "Immunological and physiological changes associated with induced positive and negative mood." *Psychosomatic Medicine, 56,* 6, 231–238.

Gallagher, R., M., Rauh, V., Haugh, L. D., Milhous, R., Callas, P. W., Langelier, R. *et al.* (1989) "Determinants of return-to-work among low back pain patients." *Pain, 39,* 55–67.

Geer, D. (1990) "Adopting a marketing orientation: Marketing made accessible to dance/movement therapists." *American Journal of Dance Therapy, 12,* 1, 45–59.

Giorgi, A. (ed.) (1985) *Phenomenology and Psychological Research.* Pittsburgh, PA: Duquesne Univeristy Press.

Gladis, M. M., Gosch, E. A., Dishuk, N. M. and Crits-Christoph, P. (1999) "Quality of life: expanding the scope of clinical significance." *Journal of Consulting and Clinical Psychology, 67,* 3, 320–31.

Glaser, R. and Kiecolt-Glaser, J. (1998) "Psychoneuroimmunology: An introduction." Paper presented at the Mind/Body Programs Symposium Series, February, Allegheny University of the Health Sciences, Philadelphia, PA.

Goff, L. C., Rebollo Pratt, R. and Madrigal, J. L. (1997) "Music listening and S-IgA levels in patients undergoing a dental procedure." *International Journal of Arts Medicine, 5,* 2, 22–6.

Goodill, S. (1992) "The journey as metaphor and method in dance/movement therapy." Paper presented at the American Dance Therapy Association 27th Annual Conference, October, Columbia, MD.

Goodill, S. (1995) *Dance/Movement Therapy for Adults with Cystic Fibrosis* (Final Report of Exploratory Research Grant Project #1-R21-RR09411-01). Bethesda, MD: National Institutes of Health, Office of Alternative Medicine.

Goodill, S. (2000a) "Nonverbal interaction between an acupuncturist and her patients: Implications for the complementary therapies." Research poster presented at the American Dance Therapy Association 35th Annual Conference, October, Seattle, WA.

Goodill, S. (2000b) "Physiological correlates of Laban described movement states: A preliminary investigation: A research proposal." Unpublished manuscript.

Goodill, S. (in press) "Research letter: Dance/movement therapy for adults with cystic fibrosis: Pilot data on mood and adherence." *Alternative Therapies in Health and Medicine.*

Goodill, S. and Morningstar, D. (1993) The role of dance/movement therapy with medically ill children. *International Journal of Arts Medicine, 2,* 24–7.

Goodman, L. S. and Holroyd, J. (1993) "Are dance/movement therapy trainees a distinctive group? Initial differences and effects of training." *American Journal of Dance Therapy, 15,* 1, 35–46.

Goodwin, P. J., Leszcz, M., Ennis, M., Koopmans, J., Vincent, L., Guther, H. *et al.* (2001) "The effect of group psychosocial support on survival in metastatic breast cancer." *The New England Journal of Medicine, 345,* 24, 1719–26.

Gorelick, K. (1989) "Metaphor the mediator: Rapprochement between the arts and psychotherapies." *The Arts in Psychotherapy: An International Journal, 16,* 149–55.

Gorham, L. and Imus, S. (1999) "Old Pain/new gains: Treatment for chronic pain patients." Paper presented at the American Dance Therapy Association 34th Annual Conference, November, Chicago, IL.

Graham-Pole, J. and Lane, M. R. (1994) "Creating an arts program in an academic medical setting." [electronic version]. *International Journal of Arts Medicine, 3,* 2, 17–26.

Green, C. J. (1985) "Psychological assessment in medical settings." In N. Schneiderman and J. Tapp (eds) *Behavioral Medicine: The Biopsychosocial Approach.* Hillsdale, NJ: Lawrence Erlbaum Associates Publishers.

Grodner, S., Braff, D., Janowsky, D. and Clopton, P. (1982) "Efficacy of art/movement therapy in elevating mood." *The Arts in Psychotherapy: An International Journal, 9,* 217–25.

Guthrie, J. (1999) "Movement and dance therapy in head injury: An evaluation." *Dance Therapy Collections, Dance Therapy Association of Australia, 2,* 24–30.

Hall, N. R., Anderson, J. A. and O'Grady, M. P. (1994) "Stress and immunity in humans: Modifying variables." In R. Glaser and J. Kiecolt-Glaser (eds) *Handbook of Human Stress and Immunity.* New York: Academic Press.

Hall, N. R. S. and O'Grady, M. P. (1991) "Psychosocial interventions and immune function." In R. Ader, D. Felton and N. Cohen (eds) *Psychoneuroimmunology* (2nd ed.). San Diego, CA: Academic Press, Inc.

Halliday, D. M., Conway, B. A., Farmer, S. F. and Rosenberg, J. R. (1998) "Using electro-encephalography to study functional coupling between cortical activity and electro-myograms during voluntary contractions in humans." *Neuroscience Letters, 241,* 1, 5–8.

Halperin, D. T. (1995) "Dancing at the edge of chaos: An ethnography of wildness and ceremony in an Afro-Brazilian possession religion." Unpublished doctoral dissertation, University of California, Berkeley, CA.

Halprin, A. (2000) *Dance as a Healing Art: Returning to Health with Movement and Imagery.* Mendocino, CA: LifeRhythm.

Hamburg, J. and Clair, A. A. (2003). "The effects of a Laban-based movement program with music on measures of balance and gait in older adults." *Activities, Adaptation and Aging, 28*, 1, 212–226.

Hanna, J. L. (1988) *Dance and Stress: Resistance, reduction and euphoria.* New York: AMS Press, Inc.

Hanna, J. L. (1995) "The power of dance: health and healing." *Journal of Alternative and Complementary Medicine, 1*, 4, 323–31.

Harpham, W. S. (1994) *After Cancer: A Guide to Your New Life.* New York: W.W. Norton and Co., Inc.

Hartman, C. R. and Burgess, A. W. (1998) "Child to child sexual abuse." *Journal of Interpersonal Violence, 3*, 4, 443–57.

Hartstein, J. (1994) "Dance/movement therapy with an HIV+ population: A pilot project." Unpublished Master's thesis, MCP Hahnemann University, Philadelphia, PA.

Hays, R. D. and Morales, L. S. (2001) "The RAND-36 measure of health-related quality of life." *Annals of Medicine, 33*, 5, 350–7.

Herbert, T. B. and Cohen, S. (1993) "Stress and immunity in humans: A meta-analytic review." *Psychosomatic Medicine, 55*, 364–79.

Higgens, L. (2001) "On the value of conducting dance/movement therapy research." *The Arts in Psychotherapy: An International Journal, 28*, 191–5.

Hill, H. (1999) "Out of the cupboard...to the brightness." *Dance Therapy Collections, Dance Therapy Association of Australia, 2*, 14–18.

Hill, H. (2003) "Dance", in Chapter 22 "Creative Care". In R. Hudson (ed.) *Dementia Nursing: A Guide to Practice.* Melbourne: Ausmed Publications.

Hiller, C. A. (1996) "Dance therapy at the Momentum AIDS Project: A study of expected outcomes for an HIV+ group." Unpublished Master's thesis, Hunter College, CUNY, New York. Abstracted in Fisher and Stark (eds) (1998) *Dance/Movement Therapy Abstracts: Doctoral Dissertations, Masters' Theses, and Special Projects, Volume 2.* Columbia, MD: Marian Chace Foundation, ADTA.

Hornyak, L. M. and Baker, E. K. (eds) (1989) *Experiential Therapies for Eating Disorders.* New York: Guilford Press.

Horrigan, B. (2000) "The importance of spirituality in mental health. An interview with David Lukoff." *Alternative Therapies in Health and Medicine, 6*, 6, 81–7.

Hughes, D. and Kleespies, P. (2001) "Suicide in the medically ill." *Suicide and Life-Threatening Behavior, 31* (supplement), 48–59.

Hunt, V. (1973) "Neuromuscular organization in emotional states." *ADTA Monograph No. 3*, 16–41.

Hyle, D. (1996) "Dance/movement therapy and body awareness exercises implemented into exercise regimen of Phase II cardiac rehabilitation patients: An experimental case study." Unpublished Master's thesis, Lesley College Graduate School of Arts and Social Sciences, Cambridge, MA. Abstracted in Fisher and Stark (eds) (1998) *Dance/Movement Therapy Abstracts: Doctoral Dissertations, Masters' Theses, and Special Projects, Volume 2.* Columbia, MD: Marian Chace Foundation, ADTA.

IAMA (International Arts Medicine Association) (2001) Newsletter, 16, 4 (December), 11.

Ireland, M. and Olson, M. (2000) "Massage therapy and therapeutic touch in children: State of the science." *Alternative Therapies in Health and Medicine, 6*, 5, 54–63.

Irwin, M. (1999) "Psychoneuroimmunology of depression: Moderators of the depression-immune link." Paper presented at the Center for Mind/Body Studies Symposium Series, February 5, MCP Hahnemann University, Philadelphia, PA.

Irwin, M., Patterson, T., Smith, T. L., Caldwell, C., Brown, S. A., Gillin, J. C. and Grant, I. (1990) "Reduction of immune function in life stress and depression." *Biological Psychiatry, 27*, 22–30.

Isselbacher, K. J., Adams, R. D., Braunwald, E., Pertersdorf, R. G. and Wilson, J. D. (1980) *Harrison's Principles of Internal Medicine* (9th ed.). New York: McGraw-Hill Book Company.

Jacobi, E. M. (1995) "The efficacy of the Bonny method of Guided Imagery and Music as experiential therapy in a primary care of persons with rheumatoid arthritis." Unpublished doctoral dissertation, The Union Institute, Cincinnati, OH.

Janco, O. (1991) "Healing in water: Dance/movement therapy in water with the chronic pain population." Unpublished Master's thesis, Antioch/New England Graduate School, Keene, NH.

Janeway, C. and Travers, P. (1996) *Immunobiology: The Immune System in Health and Disease* (2nd ed.). New York: Current Biology Ltd./Garland Publishing Inc.

Jankey, S. G. (1999) "Meaning as a factor in the quality of life of long-term care hospital residents." *Dissertation Abstracts International, 59*, 12-B, 6489.

Jasnoski, M. B. (1994) "Imagery and immunity: Implications for cancer and AIDS." Paper presented at the First Awardees Conference of the NIH-OAM, March, Bethesda, MD.

Jemmot III, J. B. (1985) "Psychoneuroimmunology: The new frontier." *American Behavioral Scientist. Special Issue: Health Psychology, 28*, 4, 497–509.

Jemmott III, J. and McClelland, D. C. (1989) "Secretory IgA as a measure of resistance to infectious disease: Comments on Stone, Cox, Valdimarsdottir, and Neale." *Behavioral Medicine* (summer), 63–71.

Johnson, D. R. (1987) "The role of the creative arts therapies in the diagnosis and treatment of psychological trauma." *The Arts in Psychotherapy: An International Journal, 14*, 1, 7–13.

Jones, B. T. (1998) "An evening with Bill T. Jones: The Marian Chace Annual Lecture and post lecture question and answer session." *American Journal of Dance Therapy, 20*, 1, 5–22.

Josephs, M. and Kasovac, N. (1999) "Movement therapy and massage therapy in a multi-disciplinary pediatric pain clinic: A biopsychosocial approach." Paper presented at the American Dance Therapy Association 34th Annual Conference, October, Chicago, IL.

Judge, J., Sandel, S., Faria, L. and Landry, N. (2002) "'We got the grant': Story of a research collaborative." Paper presented at the American Dance Therapy Association 37th Annual Conference, October, Burlington, VT.

Kaplan, R. M. (1990) "Behavior as a central outcome in health care." *American Psychologist, 45*, 11, 1211–20.

Kaplan Westbrook, B. and McKibben, H. (1989) "Dance/movement therapy with groups of outpatients with Parkinson's disease." *American Journal of Dance Therapy, 11*, 1, 27–38.

Kasovac, N. and Loman, S. (1997) "The Kestenberg Movement Profile of an infant with non-progressive myopathy post-heart transplant." Paper presented at the 32nd Annual Conference of the American Dance Therapy Association, November, Philadelphia, PA.

Katz, R. (1984) *Boiling Energy: Community Healing among the Kalahari Kung.* Boston, MA: Harvard University Press.

Kazak, A. E. (1989) "Families of chronically ill children: A systems and social-ecological model of adaptation and change" [electronic version]. *Journal of Consulting and Clinical Psychology, 57*, 1, 25–30.

Kazdin, A. E. (1982) *Single-case Research Designs.* New York: Oxford Unviersity Press.

Keenan, L. B. (1997) "Dance/movement therapy in arts medicine (S. Goodill, moderator)." Panel presentation at the American Dance Therapy Association 32nd Annual Conference, November 5–9, Philadelphia, PA.

Keller, S. E., Shiflett, S. C., Schleifer, S. J. and Bartlett, J. A. (1994) "Stress, immunity and health." In R. Glaser and J. Kiecolt-Glaser (eds) *Handbook of Human Stress and Immunity.* San Diego, CA: Academic Press.

Kemeny, M. E. (1994) "Stressful events, psychological responses and progression of HIV infection." In R. Glaser and J. M. Kiecolt-Glaser (eds) *Handbook of Human Stress and Immunity.* San Diego, CA: Academic Press.

Kestenberg, J. (1975) *Children and Parents: Psychoanalytic Studies in Development.* New York: Jason Aronson.

Kiecolt-Glaser, J. and Glaser, R. (1992) "Psychoneuroimmunology: Can psychological interventions modulate immunity?" *Journal of Consulting and Clinical Psychology, 60,* 4, 569–75.

Kierr, S. and Pilus, L. (n.d.) "Dance Movement Therapy in Rehabilitation Medicine." Unpublished manuscript.

Kierr Wise, S. (1981) "Integrating the use of music in movement therapy for patients with spinal cord injuries." *American Journal of Dance Therapy, 4,* 1, 42–51.

Kierr Wise, S. (1986) "I could have danced all night: Case studies of dance/movement therapy in rehabilitation." Unpublished manuscript.

Kleinman, A. (1973) "Some issues for a comparative study of medical healing." *International Journal of Social Psychiatry, 19,* 159–163.

Kleinman, A. and Sung, L. H. (1979) "Why do indigenous practitioners successfully heal?" *Social Sciences and Medicine, 13B,* 7–26.

Klivington, K. (1997) "Information, energy, and mind-body medicine." *ADVANCES: The Journal of Mind-Body Health, 13,* 4, 3–42.

Knapp, M. L. and Hall, J. A. (eds) (1997) *Nonverbal Communication in Human Interaction.* Fort Worth, TX: Harcourt Brace College Publishers.

Kopp, S. (1972/1988) *If You Meet the Bhudda on the Road, Kill Him!* New York: Bantam Books.

Krantz, A. (1994) "Dancing out trauma: The effects of psychophysical expression on health." Unpublished doctoral dissertation, California School of Professional Psychology, Berkeley, CA.

Krueger, D. W. and Schofield, E. (1986) "Dance/movement therapy of eating disordered patients: A model." *The Arts in Psychotherapy: An International Journal, 13,* 4, 323–31.

Kubie, L. S. (1958) *Neurotic Distortions of the Creative Process* (Vol. 22). Lawrence, KS: University of Kansas Press.

Kübler Ross, E. (1969) *On Death and Dying.* NY: Macmillan.

Kuettel, T. J. (1982) "Affective change in dance therapy." *American Journal of Dance Therapy, 5,* 56–64.

Kutz, I., Borsyenko, J. Z. and Benson, H. (1985) "Meditation and psychotherapy: A rationale for the integration of dynamic psychotherapy, the relaxation response and mindfulness meditation." *American Journal of Psychiatry, 142,* 1, 1–8.

La Greca, A. M. and Stone, W. L. (1985) "Behavioral pediatrics." In N. Schneiderman and J. Tapp (eds) *Behavioral Medicine: The Biopsychosocial Approach.* Hillsdale, NJ: Lawrence Erlbaum Associates Publishers.

Laban, R. (1980) *The Mastery of Movement.* Estover, Plymouth: Macdonald and Evans, Ltd. (Original work published 1950.)

Lazarus, R. S. (2000) "Toward better research on stress and coping." *American Psychologist, 55,* 6, 665–73.

LeDoux, J. E. (1993) "Emotional memory systems in the brain." *Behavioural Brain Research, 58,* 69–79.

Lehman, A. F. (1999) "A review of instruments for measuring quality-of-life outcomes in mental health." In N. E. Miller and K. M. Magruder (eds) *Cost-effectiveness of Psychotherapy: A Guide for Practioners, Researchers and Policymakers.* New York: Oxford University Press.

Lehrer, P. M., Sargunaraj, D. and Hochron, S. (1992) "Psychological approaches to the treatment of asthma." *Journal of Consulting and Clinical Psychology, 60,* 4, 639–43.

Leste, A. and Rust, J. (1984) "Effect of dance on anxiety." *Perceptual and Motor Skills, 58,* 767–72.

Levitan, A. A. (1999) "Oncology." In R. Temes (ed.) *Medical Hypnosis.* New York: Harcourt Brace and Co.

Levy, F. J. (1988) *Dance Movement Therapy: A Healing Art.* Reston, VA: American Alliance for Health, Physical Education and Dance.

Lewis, C. S. (1961) *A Grief Observed.* New York: Seabury Press, Inc.

Lewis, P. (1979/1994) *Theoretical Approaches in Dance/Movement Therapy.* Dubuque, IA: Kendall/Hunt Publishing Co.

Lewis, P. (2002) *Integrative Holistic Health, Healing, and Transformation: A Guide for Practitioners, Consultants, and Administrators.* Springfield, IL: Charles C. Thomas Publishers, Ltd.

Lippin, R. A. (1997) "Dance/movement therapy in arts medicine (S. Goodill, moderator)." Panel presentation at the American Dance Therapy Association 32nd Annual Conference, November 5–9, Philadelphia, PA.

Lippin, R. A. (1980) "Dance of Alchemy." *The Arts in Psychotherapy: An International Journal, 7,* 4, 273–4.

Lobel, M. and Dunkel-Schetter, C. (1990) "Conceptualizing stress to study effects on health: Environmental, perceptual, and emotional components." *Anxiety Research, 3,* 213–30.

Loewy, J. V. (ed.) (1997) *Music Therapy and Pediatric Pain.* Cherry Hill, NJ: Jeffrey Books.

Loman, S. and Foley, L. (1996) "Models for understanding the nonverbal process in relationships." *The Arts in Psychotherapy: An International Journal, 23,* 4, 341–50.

Lotan, N. and Yirmiya, N. (2002) "Body movement, presence of parents and the process of falling asleep in toddlers." *International Journal of Behavioral Development, 26,* 1, 81–8.

Lotan-Mesika, S. (2000) "A dance/movement therapy support group model for young siblings of children with cancer: A theoretical model." Unpublished Master's thesis, MCP Hahnemann University, Philadelphia, PA.

Loughlin, E. E. (1993) "'Why was I born among mirrors?' Therapeutic dance for teenage girls and women with Turner Syndrome." *American Journal of Dance Therapy, 15,* 2, 107–24.

Lowen, A. (1976) *Bioenergetics.* New York: Penguin Books.

Lukoff, D., Edwards, D. and Miller, M. (1998) "The case study as a scientific method for researching alternative therapies." *Alternative Therapies in Health and Medicine, 4,* 2, 44–52.

Lynch, J. J. (1977) *The Broken Heart.* New York: Basic Books.

Lynn-McHale, D. J. and Deatrick, J. A. (2000) "Trust between family and health care provider" [electronic version]. *Journal of Family Nursing, 6,* 3, 210–30.

Malchiodi, C. A. (1993) "Medical art therapy: Contributions to the field of arts medicine" [electronic version]. *International Journal of Arts Medicine, 2*, 2, 28–32.

Malchiodi, C. A. (ed.) (1999a) *Medical Art Therapy with Adults.* London: Jessica Kingsley Publishers.

Malchiodi, C. A. (ed.) (1999b) *Medical Art Therapy with Children.* London: Jessica Kingsley Publishers.

Mancarella, K. M. (2000) "A dance/movement therapy support group model for children of cancer patients." Unpublished Master's thesis, MCP Hahnemann University, Philadelphia, PA.

Mannheim, E. (2000) "Dancetherapie in the oncological rehabilitation: Results to the effects of quality of life" [English abstract obtained from the author]. *Zeitschrift Für Musik-, Tanz- und Kunsttherapie, 11*, 2, 80–6.

Massie, M. J., Holland, J. C. and Straker, N. (1989) "Psychotherapeutic interventions." In J. C. Holland and J. H. Rowland (eds) *Handbook of Psychooncology: Psychological Care of the Patient with Cancer.* New York: Oxford University Press.

Matthews, D. A., McCullough, M. E., Larson, D. B., Koenig, H. G., Swyers, J. P. and Greenwald Milano, M. (1998) "Religious commitment and health status: A review of the research and implications for family medicine." *Archives of Family Medicine, 7*, 118–24.

McCullough, M. E., Hoyt, W. T., Larson, D. B., Koenig, H. G. and Thoresen, C. (2000) "Religious involvement and mortality: A meta-analytic review." *Health Psychology, 19*, 3, 211–22.

McDonough, A. L. (2001) *Labview: Data acquisition and Analysis for the Movement Sciences.* Upper Saddle River, NJ: Prentice-Hall, Inc.

McKinley, E. D. (2000) "Under toad fays: Surviving the uncertainty of cancer recurrence." *Annals of Internal Medicine, 133*, 6, 479–80.

McKinney, C. H., Antoni, M. H., Kumar, M. and Tims, F. C. (1997) "Effects of guided imagery and music (GIM) therapy on mood and cortisol in healthy adults." *Health Psychology, 16*, 390–400.

McWhinney, I. R., Epstein, R. M. and Freeman, T. R. (1997) "Rethinking somatization." *Annals of Internal Medicine, 126*, 9, 747–50.

Melsom, A. M. (1999) "Dance/movement therapy for psychosocial aspects of heart disease and cancer: An exploratory literature review." Unpublished Master's thesis, MCP Hahnemann University, Philadelphia, PA.

Melzak, R. (1999) "From the gate to the neuromatrix." *Pain*, Supplement, *6* (August) S121–6.

Mendelsohn, J. (1999) "Dance/movement therapy for hospitalized children." *American Journal of Dance Therapy, 21*, 2, 65–80.

Micozzi, M. S. (1997) "Fundamentals of complementary and alternative medicine." Paper presented at the Mind/Body Programs Symposium Series, February, Allegheny University of the Health Sciences, Philadelphia, PA.

Moerman, D. E. and Jonas, W. B. (2002) "Deconstructing the placebo effect and finding the meaning response." *Annals of Internal Medicine, 136*, 471–6.

Monroe, S. M. (1989) "Stress and social support." In N. Schneiderman, S. Weiss and P. Kaufmann (eds) *Handbook of Research Methods in Cardiovascular Behavioral Medicine.* New York: Plenum Press.

Montagu, A. (1971) *Touching: The Human Significance of the Skin.* New York: Columbia University Press.

Montello, L. (1996) "Arts Medicine editorial." *International Journal of Arts Medicine, 5*, 2, 44–5.

Morgan, D. L. and Morgan, R. K. (2001) "Single-participant research design." *American Psychologist, 56*, 2, 119–27.

Moss, S. and Anolik, S. (1984) "The use of skin temperature biofeedback to facilitate relaxation training for retarded adults: A pilot study." *American Journal of Dance Therapy, 7*, 49–57.

Moyers, B. (1993) *Healing and the Mind.* New York: Doubleday.

Mrazek, D. A. and Klinnert, M. (1991) "Asthma: Psychoneuroimmunologic considerations." In R. Ader, D. Felton and N. Cohen (eds) *Psychoneuroimmunology* (2nd ed). San Diego, CA: Academic Press, Inc.

Murphy, C. R. (1988) "COPD: Exercise, psychological support and education." In L. K. Hall (ed.) *Epidemiology, Behavior, Change and Intervention in Chronic Disease.* Champagne, IL: Life Enhancement Publishers.

Murphy, P. (1985) "Studies of loss and grief: Tragic opportunities for growth." *The American Journal of Hospice Care,* March/April, 10–14.

Nachmanovich, S. (1990) *Free Play: Improvisation in Life and Arts.* New York: Penguin Putnam, Inc.

National Institutes of Health (NIH) National Center for Complementory and Alternative Medicine (n.d.) "'What is CAM?'" Retrieved March 10, 2004 from the World Wide Web: www.nccam.nih.gov/health/whatiscam

National Institutes of Health (NIH) National Center for Complementary and Alternative medicine (2001) "National conference explores the basis for and potential application of the placebo effect" NIH NCCAM *Newsletter, 3*, 1, 1.

Navarre, D. (1982) "Posture sharing in dyadic interaction." *American Journal of Dance Therapy, 5*, 28–42.

Nelson, C. J., Rosenfeld, B., Breitbart, W. and Galietta, M. (2002) "Spirituality, religion and depression in the terminally ill." *Psychosomatics, 43*, 3, 213–20.

Neuman-Bluestein, D. (1999) "You gotta have heart: Integrating dance therapy into cardiac rehabilitation stress management." Paper presented at the American Dance Therapy Association 34th Annual Conference, October, Chicago, IL.

Newman, M. C., Lorico, A., Goodill, S., Cheley, L. and Minassian, S. (2000) "Listening to our patients: The experience of women with PCOS undergoing acupuncture for anovulation." Paper presented at the Society of Teachers of Family Medicine, Northeast Regional Meeting, October, Philadelphia, PA.

North, M. (1972) *Personality Assessment through Movement.* London: MacDonald and Evans, Ltd.

Pallaro, P. (1993) "Culture, self and body-self." In Bejjani, F. J. (ed.) *Current Research in Arts Medicine.* Chicago, IL: a cappella books.

Pallaro, P. (1994) "Somatic countertransference: The therapist in relationship." Paper presented at the Third European Arts Therapies Conference of the European Consortium for Arts Therapies Education, September, University of Ferrara, Italy.

Pallaro, P. (ed.) (1999) *Authentic Movement: Essays by Mary Starks Whitehouse, Janet Adler and Joan Chodorow.* London: Jessica Kingsley Publishers.

Palmer, J. and Leniart, K. (eds) (2003) *Report on the Arts in Healthcare Symposium* Washington, DC: Society for the Arts in Healthcare.

Parham, P. (2000) *The Immune System.* New York: Garland Publishing/Taylor and Francis Group.

Parkinson's Disease Foundation (2004) "Motivating moves for people with Parkinson's." Retrieved April 25, 2004, from the World Wide Web: www.pdf.org

Pennebaker, J. (2000) "Traumatic experience, disclosure, and physical health." Paper presented at the Mind/Body Programs Symposium Series, April, MCP Hahnemann University, Philadelphia, PA.

Pennebaker, J., Kiecolt-Glaser, J. and Glaser, R. (1988) "Disclosure of traumas and immune function: Health implications for psychotherapy." *Journal of Consulting Psychology, 56*, 239–45.

Perowsky, G. (1991) "Working with pain: A self study." *American Journal of Dance Therapy, 13*, 1, 49–58.

Perrin, K. O. (2001) "How do intensive care unit (ICU) nurses interact with physicians to facilitate discussion of patients' preferences about resuscitation?" Unpublished doctoral dissertation, The Union Institute, Cincinnati, OH.

Pert, C. B. (1997) *Molecules of Emotion: Why You Feel the Way You Feel.* New York: Scribner.

Pert, C. B., Ruff, M. R., Weber, R. J. and Herkenham, M. (1985) "Neuropeptides and their receptors: A psychosomatic network." *Journal of Immunology, 135*, 2, 820s–826s.

Petrone, K. (1997) "The role of dance/movement therapy in a cancer support group: A group case study." Unpublished Master's thesis, MCP Hahnemann University, Philadelphia, PA.

Pfifferling, J.-H. and Gilley, K. (2000) "Overcoming compassion fatigue." *Family Practice Management,* April, 39–44.

Pfurtscheller, G. and Neuper, C. (1997) "Motor imagery activates primary sensorimotor area in humans." *Neuroscience Letters, 239,* 2–3, 65–8.

Pilisuk, M., Wentzel, P., Barry, O. and Tennant, J. (1997) "Participant assessment of a nonmedical breast cancer support group." *Alternative Therapies in Health and Medicine, 3,* 5, 72–80.

Prugh, D. (1983) "Reactions of children and families to hospitalization and medical and surgical procedures." In D. Prugh (ed.) *Psychological Aspects of Pediatrics.* Philadelphia, PA: Lea and Ferbiger.

Pylvänäinen, P. (2003). "Body image: A tripartite model for use in dance/movement therapy." *American Journal of Dance Therapy, 25,* 1, 39–55.

Rabin, B. S., Kusnecov, A., Shurin, M., Zhou, D. and Rasnick, S. (1994) "Mechanistic aspects of stressor-induced immune alteration." In R. Glaser and J. M. Kiecolt-Glaser (eds) *Handbook of Human Stress and Immunity.* San Diego, CA: Academic Press.

Reibel, D. K., Greeson, J. M., Brainard, G. C. and Rosenzweig, S. (2001) "Mindfulness-based stress reduction and health-related quality of life in a heterogeneous patient population." *General Hospital Psychiatry, 23,* 4, 183–92.

Revenson, T. A. (1994) "Social support and marital coping with chronic illness." *Annals of Behavioral Medicine, 16,* 2, 122–30.

Richardson, M. A., Post-White, J., Grimm, E.A., Moye, L.A., Singletary, S.E., and Justice, B. (1997) "Coping, life attitudes, and immune responses to imagery and group support after breast cancer treatment." *Alternative Therapies in Health and Medicine, 3,* 5, 62–70.

Rider, M. L. (1995) "The prospective role of movement therapy in holistic mind/body medicine: As exemplified by its application with the cancer population." Unpublished Master's thesis, University of California, Los Angeles, CA.

Ritter, M. and Low, K. G. (1996) "Effects of dance/movement therapy: A meta-analysis." *The Arts in Psychotherapy: An International Journal, 23,* 3, 249–60.

Rodenhauser, P. (1996) "On creativity and medicine." *The Pharos* (fall), 2–6.

Rossi, E. L. (1993) *The Psychobiology of Mind–Body Healing* (revised ed.). New York and London: W.W. Norton and Co.

Rossi, E. L. (1999) "An introduction to clinical hypnosis and mind/body healing: A psychobiological approach to the hypnotherapeutic arts (3-day course with Institute Certificate)." Course given at The Psychology of Consciousness, Energy Medicine and Dynamic Change, 3rd International Conference of The National Institute for the Clinical Application of Behavioral Medicine, Hilton Head, SC.

Rossman, M. L. (2000) *Guided Imagery for Self Healing* (2nd ed.). Tiburon, CA: H.J. Kramer.

Russell, M. L. (1996) "The use of dance/movement based support groups to address occupational stress among pediatric nurses." Unpublished Master's thesis, MCP Hahnemann University, Philadelphia, PA.

Sackler, A. M. (1984) Lecture delivered at Hahnemann University, Philadelphia. April 26.

Sakamoto, M. (2001) "The effect of the combination of movement and guided-imagery among depressed university students: A psychophysiological study." Unpublished Master's thesis, MCP Hahnemann University, Philadelphia, PA.

Salovey, P., Detweiler, J. B., Steward, W. T. and Rothman, A. J. (2000) "Emotional states and physical health" [electronic version]. *American Psychologist, 55,* 1, 110–21.

Sandel, S. (1993a) "Imagery in dance therapy groups: A developmental approach." In S. Sandel, S. Chaiklin and A. Lohn (eds) *Foundations of Dance/Movement Therapy: The Life and Work of Marian Chace.* Columbia, MD: American Dance Therapy Association.

Sandel, S. (1993b) "The process of empathic reflection in dance therapy." In S. Sandel, S. Chaiklin and A. Lohn (eds) *The Foundations of Dance/Movement Therapy: The Life and Work of Marian Chace.* Columbia, MD: American Dance Therapy Association.

Sandel, S., Chaiklin, S. and Lohn, A. (eds) (1993) *Foundations of Dance/Movement Therapy: The Life and Work of Marian Chace.* Columbia, MD: American Dance Therapy Association.

Schalkwijk-Vanderkruk, M. E. (1993) "Educational interventions in dance/movement therapy with chronic pain patients." Unpublished Master's thesis, Goucher College, Towson, MD. Abstracted in Fisher and Stark (eds) (1998) *Dance/Movement Therapy Abstracts: Doctoral Dissertations, Masters' Theses, and Special Projects, Volume 2.* Columbia, MD: Marian Chace Foundation, ADTA.

Scheflen, A. (1982) "Comments on the significance of interaction rhythms." In M. Davis (ed.) *Interaction Rhythms.* New York: Human Science Press.

Scheflen, A. with Scheflen, A. (1972) *Body Language and the Social Order.* Englewood Cliffs, NJ: Prentice-Hall, Inc.

Schilder, P. (1950) *The Image and Appearance of the Human Body.* New York: International Universities Press, Inc.

Schmais, C. (1974) "Dance therapy in perspective." In K. C. Mason (ed.) *Focus on Dance VII: Dance Therapy.* Washington, DC: AAHPERD/NEA.

Schmais, C. (1985) "Healing processes in dance therapy." *American Journal of Dance Therapy, 8,* 17–36.

Schneiderman, L. and Baum, A. (1991) "Acute and chronic stress and the immune system." In N. Schneiderman, P. McCabe and A. Baum (eds) *Perspectives in Behavioral Medicine: Stress and Disease Processes.* Hillsdale, NJ: Lawrence Erlbaum.

Schneiderman, N., Antoni, M., Ironson, G., Klimas, N., LaPerriere, Kumar, M., Esterling, B. and Fletcher, M. A. (1994) "HIV-1, immunity and behavior." In R. Glaser and J. M. Kiecolt-Glaser (eds) *Handbook of Human Stress and Immunity.* San Diego, CA: Academic Press.

Schneiderman, N. and McCabe, P. M. (1989) "Psychophysiologic strategies in laboratory research." In N. Schneiderman, S. Weiss and P. Kaufman (eds) *Handbook of Research Methods in Cardiovascular Behavioral Medicine.* New York: Plenum Press.

Schonwetter, R. S., Hawke, W. and Knight, C. F. (eds) (1999) *Hospice and Palliative Medicine: Core Curriculum and Review Syllabus.* Dubuque, IA: Kendall/Hunt Publishing Co.

Schwartz, G. (1982) "Testing the biopsychosocial model: The ultimate challenge facing behavioral medicine?" *Journal of Consulting and Clinical Psychology, 50,* 6, 1040–53.

Schwartz, G. and Russek, L. G. S. (2001) "Parental love and health: Russek and Schwartz." In H. Dienstfrey (ed.) "An Advances forum: The state of the science: The best evidence for the involvement of thought and feelings in physical health" [feature article]. *Advances in Mind–Body Medicine, 17,* 2–59.

Seibel, J. (2001) "Review of the book *Dance as a Healing Art, Returning to Health with Movement and Imagery*". *American Journal of Dance Therapy, 23,* 45–6.

Seides, M. (1986) "Dance/movement therapy as a modality in the treatment of the psychosocial complications of heart disease." *American Journal of Dance Therapy, 9,* 83–101.

Selye, H. (1956/1976) *The Stress of Life* (revised ed.). New York: McGraw-Hill Book Company.

Serlin, I. A. (1993) "Root images of healing in dance therapy." *American Journal of Dance Therapy, 15,* 65–76.

Serlin, I. A. (1996a) "Interview with Anna Halprin." *American Journal of Dance Therapy, 18,* 115–24.

Serlin, I. A. (1996b) "Kinaesthetic imagining." *Journal of Humanistic Psychology, 36,* 25–33.

Serlin, I. A. (1999a) "Arts medicine in a complementary medicine setting using dance/movement therapy with women with breast cancer." Paper presented at the American Dance Therapy Association 34th Annual Conference, October Chicago, IL.

Serlin, I. A. (1999b) "Imagery, movement and breast cancer." In C. C. Clark and R. J. Gordon (eds) *Encyclopedia of Complementary Health Practice.* New York: Springer Publishing Co.

Serlin, I. A. (2001) *Dance Therapy* [videotape]. Co-produced by the Marian Chace Foundation of the American Dance Therapy Association. Available from the American Psychological Association, 750 First Street, NE, Washington, DC 20002.

Serlin, I. A., Classen, C., Frances, B. and Angell, K. (2000) "Symposium: Support groups for women with breast cancer: Traditional and alternative expressive approaches." *The Arts in Psychotherapy: An International Journal, 27,* 123–38.

Shapiro, A. I. (1999) *The Movement Phrase and its Clinical Significance in Dance/Movement Therapy.* Unpublished Master's thesis, MCP Hahnemann University, Philadelphia, PA.

Sherwood, L. (1997) *Human Physiology: From Cells to Systems* (3rd ed.). Belmont, CA: Wadsworth Publishing Co.

Siegel, K., Karus, D. and Raveis, V. (1996) "Adjustment of children facing the death of a parent due to cancer" [electronic version]. *Journal of the American Academy of Child and Adolescent Psychiatry, 35,* 442–50.

Silberman-Deihl, L. and Komisaruk, B. R. (1985) "Treating psychogenic somatic disorders through body metaphor." *American Journal of Dance Therapy, 8,* 37–45.

Simon, H. B. (1991) "Exercise and human immune function." In R. Ader, D. Felton and N. Cohen (eds) *Psychoneuroimmunology* (2nd ed.). San Diego, CA: Academic Press, Inc.

Singh, B., Berman, B., Hadhasy, V. and Creamer, P. (1998) "A pilot study of cognitive behavioral therapy in fibromyalgia." *Alternative Therapies in Health and Medicine, 4,* 2, 67–70.

Smith, K. W., Avis, N. E. and Assmann, S. F. (1999) "Distinguishing between quality of life and health status in quality of life research: A meta-analysis." *Quality of Life Research: An International Journal of Quality of Life Aspects of Treatment, Care and Rehabilitation, 8*, 447–59.

Smith, R. C. (2001) "An evidence base for identifying patients' thoughts and feelings." In H. Dienstfrey (ed.) "An Advances forum: The state of the science: The best evidence for the involvement of thought and feelings in physical health" [feature article]. *Advances in Mind–Body Medicine, 17*, 31–4.

Smith, T. W. and Nicassio, P. M. (1995) "Psychological practice: Clinical application of the biopsychosocial model." In P. M. Nicassio and T. W. Smith (eds) *Managing Chronic Illness: A Biopsychosocial Perspective.* Washington, DC: American Psychological Association.

Sobel, D. S. (1995) "Rethinking medicine: Improving health outcomes with cost-effective psychosocial interventions." *Psychosomatic Medicine, 57*, 234–44.

Somerfield, M. R. and McCrae, R. R. (2000) "Stress and coping research: Methodological challenges, theoretical advances, and clinical applications." *American Psychologist, 55*, 6, 620–5.

Spiegel, D. (2001) "Mind matters—Group therapy and survival in breast cancer." [editorial]. *New England Journal of Medicine, 345*, 24, 1767–8.

Spiegel, D., Bloom, J., Kraemer, H. and Gottheil, E. (1989) "Effect of psychosocial treatment on survival of patients with metastatic breast cancer." *Lancet*, October 14 (8668), 888–91.

Spiegel, D., Bloom, J. and Yalom, I. D. (1981) "Group support for patients with metastatic breast cancer." *Archives of General Psychiatry, 38*, 527–33.

Spira, J. (1997) "Understanding and developing psychotherapy groups for medically ill patients." In J. Spira (ed.) *Group Therapy for Medically Ill Patients.* New York: The Guilford Press.

Stern, D. (1977) *The First Relationship: Infant and Mother.* Cambridge, MA: Harvard University Press.

Stern, D. (1990) *Diary of a Baby.* New York: Basic Books.

Stewart, N. J., McMullen, L. M. and Rubin, L. D. (1994) "Movement therapy with depressed inpatients: A randomized multiple single case design." *Archives of Psychiatric Nursing, 8*, 1, 22–9.

Stone, A. A., Cox, D. S., Valdimarsdottir, H. and Neale, J. M. (1987) "Secretory IgA as a measure of immunocompetence." *Journal of Human Stress, 13*, fall, 136–40.

Streepay, J. and Gross, M. M. (1998) "Influence of emotional intent on dance kinematics." Paper presented at the NACOB '98, The Third North American Congress on Biomechanics, August, Waterloo, Canada.

Summer, L. (1990) *Guided Imagery and Music in the Institutional Setting* (2nd ed.). St. Louis, MO: MMB Music, Inc.

Tapp, J. and Warner, R. (1985) "The multisystems view of health and disease." In N. Schneiderman and J. Tapp (eds) *Behavioral Medicine: The Biopsychosocial Approach.* Hillsdale, NJ: Lawrence Erlbaum Associates Publishers.

Tashakkori, A. and Teddlie, C. (1998) *Mixed Methodology: Combining Qualitative and Quantitative Approaches.* Thousand Oaks, CA: Sage Publications.

Tatum-Fairfax, A. (2002) "Health, treatment and imagery of gout pain." Unpublished manuscript, MCP Hahnemann University, Philadelphia, PA.

Taylor, E. (2000) "Mind–body medicine and alternative therapies at Harvard: Is this the reintroduction of psychology into general medical practice?" *Alternative Therapies in Health and Medicine, 6*, 6, 32–3.

Taylor, S. (1990) "Health psychology: The science and the field." *American Psychologist, 45,* 1, 40–50.

Taylor, S. E., Kemeny, M. E., Bower, J. E., Gruenewald, T. L. and Reed, G. M. (2000) "Psychological resources, positive illusions, and health" [electronic version]. *American Psychologist, 55,* 1, 99–109.

Temes, R. (1999) "Welcome to hypnosis." In R. Temes (ed.) *Medical Hypnosis.* New York: Harcourt Brace and Co.

Thulin, K. (1997) "When words are not enough: Dance therapy as a method of treatment for patients with psychsomatic disorders." *American Journal of Dance Therapy, 19,* 1, 25–43.

Turk, D. C. and Meichenbaum, D. (1988) "Adherence to self-care regimens: The patient's perspective." In J. J. Sweet, R. H. Rozensky and S. M. Tovian (eds) *Handbook of Clinical Psychology in Medical Settings.* New York: Plenum Press.

Turner, J. A., Deyo, R. A., Loeser, J. D., Von Korff, M. and Fordyce, W. E. (1994) "The importance of placebo effects in pain treatment and research." *Journal of the American Medical Association, 271,* 1609–14.

Turner, V. (1967) "Betwixt and between: The liminal period in rites of passage." In L. C. Mahdi, S. Foster. and M. Little (eds) *Betwixt and Between: Patterns of Masculine and Feminine Initiation.* La Salle, IL: Open Court.

Vaillant, G. E. (2000) "Adaptive mental mechanisms: Their role in a positive psychology" [electronic version]. *American Psychologist, 55,* 1, 89–98.

Vamos, M. (1993). "Body image in chronic illness – A reconceptualization." *International Journal of Psychiatry in Medicine, 23,* 2, 163–78.

Verghese, J., Lipton, R. B., Katz, M. J., Hall, C. B., Derby, C. A., Kuslansky, G., Ambrose, A. F., Swilinski, M. and Buschke, H. (2003) "Leisure activities and the risk of dementia in the elderly." *The New England Journal of Medicine, 348,* 2508–2516.

Wadsworth Hervey, L. (2000) *Artistic Inquiry in Dance/Movement Therapy: Creative Alternatives for Research.* New York: Charles C. Thomas Publishers.

Wagaman, M. J. (1999) "Hypnosis and its usefulness in managing patients with respiratory problems." In R. Temes (ed.) *Medical Hypnosis.* New York: Harcourt Brace and Co.

Wallace, J. (2000) "The use of dance/movement therapy with a chronic pain population. Research poster session abstracts from the 1999 and 2000 conferences." *American Journal of Dance Therapy, 22,* 2, 130.

Warner, R. (1985) "Communication in health care." In N. Schneiderman and J. Tapp (eds) *Behavioral Medicine: The Biopsychosocial Approach.* Hillsdale, N.J.: Lawrence Erlbaum Associates Publishers.

Watson, A. (2001) "Rhythm as a therapeutic factor: A qualitative case analysis of a traditional healing ceremony among the Bambara of West Africa, with implications for dance/movement therapy." Unpublished Master's thesis, MCP Hahnemann University, Philadelphia, PA.

Watts-Jones, D. (1990) "Toward a stress scale for African–American women." *Psychology of Women Quarterly, 14,* 271–5.

Westwood, G. (1995) "Dance/movement therapy: A vital adjunctive treatment for person living with AIDS: A catalyst for change." Unpublished Master's thesis, Naropa Institute, Boulder, CO. Abstracted in Fisher and Stark (eds) (1998) *Dance/Movement Therapy Abstracts: Doctoral Dissertations, Masters' Theses, and Special Projects, Volume 2.* Columbia, MD: Marian Chace Foundation, ADTA.

Whitehouse, W., Digges, D.F., Orne, E.C., Keller, S.E., Bates, B.L., Bauer, N.K. *et al.* (1996) "Psychosocial and immune effects of self-hypnosis training for stress management throughout the first semester of medical school." *Psychosomatic Medicine, 58,* 249–63.

Wickramasekera, I. (1998) "Secrets kept from the mind but not the body or behavior: The unsolved problems of identifying and treating somatization and psychophysiological disease." *Advances in Mind–Body Medicine, 14,* 81–132.

Winnicott, D. W. (1971/1985) *Playing and Reality.* London: Northcote House.

Winstead-Fry, P. and Kijek, J. (1999) "An integrative review and meta-analysis of therapeutic touch research." *Alternative Therapies in Health and Medicine, 5,* 58–67.

Winters, R. and Anderson, J. B. (1985) "The neurologic bases of behavior." In N. Schneiderman and J. Tapp (eds) *Behavioral Medicine: The Biopsychosocial Approach.* Hillsdale, NJ: Lawrence Erlbaum Associates Publishers.

Wise, J. K. and Kierr Wise, S. (1985) *The Overeaters.* New York: Human Sciences Press.

Yalom, I. D. (1995) *The Theory and Practice of Group Psychotherapy* (4th ed.). New York: Basic Books.

Yapko, M. D. (1990) *Trancework: An Introduction to the Practice of Clinical Hypnosis* (2nd ed.). Bristol, PA: Brunner/Mazel.

Yardley, L. (1996) "Reconciling discursive and materialist perspectives on health and illness: A reconstruction of the biopsychosocial approach." *Theory and Psychology, 6,* 3, 485–508.

Yuval, M. (1997) "'A Dance for Life': Dance/movement therapy with pediatric oncology patients." Paper presented at the American Dance Therapy Association 32nd Annual Conference, Philadelphia, PA.

Zacharias, J. (1984) "Panel presentation." In "Looking ahead, planning together: The creative arts in therapy as an integral part of treatment for the 90's." Proceedings from a symposium sponsored by the Creative Arts in Therapy Program, June, Hahnemann University, Philadelphia.

Subject Index

Dance and movement therapy is referred to as DMT throughout the index

Author Index